The author is 55 years old, and married with 3 sons, 3 grandchildren, and a Jack Russell.

Jane has been writing freelance for quite a few years for various greeting card companies. She loves reading, watching horror films, enjoys gardening, hates cooking and Cornwall is her favourite place.

LOSING DIANA

I dedicate my book to my niece and nephew. I am so proud of them for looking after their mum so well during her illness. I thank my husband for being there every step of the way. My dear mum, without her help life would have been much harder. Thank you to all the people involved in the care of Diana, especially her two favourite carers. My sons and their partners for all their support and friends and neighbours for being the best.

Jane Benham

LOSING DIANA

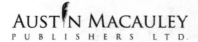
AUSTIN MACAULEY
PUBLISHERS LTD.

A CIP catalogue record for this title is available from the British Library.

ISBN 978 184963 481 6

www.austinmacauley.com

First Published (2014)
Austin Macauley Publishers Ltd.
25 Canada Square
Canary Wharf
London
E14 5LB

Printed and bound in Great Britain

Chapter 1

There is one date in my life I will never forget and that date is 6th March, it was the day my sister got married in 1982 and the day she died in 2010. The happiest day of her life and the saddest day of mine.

At the age of forty-nine she lost her life to one of the most terrible diseases ever, Motor Neurone. Fortunately she was never aware of what she had as at exactly the same time the consultant diagnosed Dementia; a double cruel blow! The Dementia saved her the heartbreak of knowing that she wouldn't survive this terrible disease, leaving behind all the people that were so special to her and more importantly her two children. My family and I lived every second of it with her; her deterioration that seemed to speed on its way with no time to take a breath.

I can't begin to tell you the shockwaves it sent through my body as we were given her diagnoses. Sat in the small insignificant room, while the consultant quietly gave us his findings.

I always believed my family were invincible and that we were good people; if you're good and kind bad things don't happen! But oh, yes they do.

If it isn't about being kind or good or even luck, then it must be fate; it was my sister's fate that at forty-nine it was her destiny to die.

That is what I now believe.

All of our lives have changed. You're happily or maybe not happily walking along one path and then bang! You're forced to take another one. Has it changed me? Yes, it definitely has; I scrutinise more and ask questions more, I like being in my own home, my safe place. I suppose I worry more; no, I definitely worry more.

I'm different inside but try to appear the same on the outside, so as not to worry the people I care for, because they all went through the same as me.

I decided to write this book because of everything we went through with Diana. And it has been my saviour while I tried to get my head around all that we were going through. Even though my sister wasn't famous and hadn't done anything outstanding, (although giving birth is pretty outstanding!) she hadn't climbed a mountain, or sailed around the world; she meant so much to us as a family. She was a wonderful mum, a good person, a loving daughter, a favourite aunty, my kind beautiful sister and my best friend. I wanted to dedicate this book to her two children Liam and Lauren who have not only suffered from their father leaving them, they also had to watch their mother's terrible illness take her a little further away from them day by day. Their courage has been truly amazing especially for such young people; also my nephew Liam copes with learning disabilities every single day of his life. We are just ordinary people who have had to cope as best we could with Diana's devastating illness. It has been a journey of heartache, inner strength, determination and love.

I now believe people are stronger than they ever believed possible. I have been tested to where I felt like walking out and leaving so many problems behind, but I didn't and I couldn't because they are my family. And I'm not the type to desert a sinking ship! Because, oh, boy at times that's what it felt like.

When something like this happens there are those few special people that are there for you, lifting you up when it gets tough.

When I have told people the story they are in disbelief that we had so much to cope with, especially the awful situation my niece and nephew found themselves left in. Because it is such a story I decided to write it down as a tribute to my sister, her children and our family. To tell the whole story from start to finish and what happened in between to my family.

Unbelievable, very painful, extremely sad, but with sheer determination we all came through it.

31st October 2007; a date etched in my brain forever! The awful day Diana's husband walked out on her. She went into complete meltdown, he was the love of her life, she became a different person overnight. From then on we became the people she turned to, she could cope with nothing. Her two children became her carers, me and my mum supporting them as much as we could.

The one thing she wanted we couldn't give her and that was her husband to come back. It was such an awful situation to be in. I felt so sorry for her and angry at him, he did come back for a while I think because he missed his children, but he refused to stop seeing his girlfriend. He went again on 10th December 2007.

Her two children had known about the problems between their parents long before I did, Diana had asked them to keep it to themselves, she was hoping that the affair would blow over and the rest of her family would never need to know.

But I knew something had been wrong with Diana in spring of 2007. She had altered so much, she had lost the sparkle in her eyes and she seemed preoccupied with something. And she had lost a little weight. She came to my house as normal most days for a cup of tea, once the children had left for school, she chatted on as normal about things, like the programmes we had watched on the TV the night before. We talked as we always did about our children and what they had been up to, how school was going, but what I noticed was the lack of enthusiasm in her voice; it had a sadness to it. She seemed to me she was going through the motions. I couldn't put my finger on it but she was just different; there but not the same. She was always a smart person but she seemed to take more care with her makeup and her wardrobe seemed to double in size as everyday she wore a new outfit. I can't even remember what day I first noticed her change as it was so gradual. I wish then that I had asked her if something was troubling her but I'm ashamed to say I didn't. The vibes she gave off almost warned me not to ask her. It is difficult to explain but it was like she didn't want me to ask. Diana was never one to keep a secret, so if she wanted to keep this one to herself then it wasn't my place to ask.

In fact I felt too scared to ask. Deep down I felt it was something awful but she wasn't ready to share with any of us, so I carried on as normal while I waited.

My own life had been so much quieter and less hectic since my youngest had become more independent. Adam my husband and I had more time to ourselves. We had joined the National Trust, enjoying our days out and each other's company. I especially loved the gardens of the many Houses we visited. My own garden is tiny and it always made me wish our garden was larger so that I could have all the incredible plants and flowers we came across. The Houses didn't fascinate me as much as they did Adam, although the architecture of the Houses was always so impressive. Adam loves history and is very knowledgeable because of it. He enjoyed looking at the old furniture, studying the portraits and meticulously exploring every nook and cranny in the grand rooms. He seemed to know what questions to ask the Trust's volunteers dotted around. I remember one such person asking what I liked in one particular room. I felt such a fool when I replied that the ceiling looked nice, it sounded so dumb. After that I avoided any intelligent looking person with a clipboard!

I prefer places where I know a bit about the owner like Jane Austin's house in Chawton – now that is fascinating. I could spend hours there, I love her work.

The highlight for me was to see in the flesh the little table where she wrote her wonderful novels; the fantastic *Pride and Prejudice*, I don't know of anyone not in love with Mr Darcy!! Now there I could ask questions because I knew about Jane Austen, her life and her novels.

But wherever we went I enjoyed it and the freedom, and the unhurried days out. And I counted myself lucky I didn't have to cook Sunday dinner, in fact I was spoiled rotten by Adam.

I must admit we have travelled many miles just to find somewhere different to visit. We'd just make a decision and go!

We get on very well and laugh at the same things. I enjoy his company, he is so easy going and I couldn't imagine life without him. Soppy? Yeah.

We had our first holiday on our own without the kids' cries of, 'I'm bored, I need a wee, I'm starving, I feel sick, he's looking at me,' meaning a sibling was beginning to annoy the others! And of course the famous, 'are we there yet?' It's amazing what a child can come up with once bored on a journey longer than usual.

The car is so much lighter now, as like most mums everything that may be needed on these journeys is packed: drinks, wet wipes for sticky fingers, food for hungry tummies, plastic bag in case anyone wants to throw up, even an empty lemonade bottle in case an urgent wee is needed, (obviously only applying to boys). All that sat on our car's back seat now was one large shared suitcase and a small box of essentials once we reached our destination.

It was just how I imagined our first taste of freedom was going to be, and I couldn't think of one thing that could change it, but how wrong was I?

We watched our sons play football at the weekend; we had the odd takeaway and DVD to watch, usually a horror. (I love horrors!) So I was as happy as could be with my quiet uninteresting life, but one person's actions took that away from us.

And changed my niece and nephew's lives forever!

Adam and I had gone Christmas shopping at a shopping centre in Basingstoke. We had bought most of the Christmas presents. It didn't take long as I always go with a list, as shopping is my least favourite thing in the world, second to cooking. We stopped at a little café to eat, me with burger and chips already planning my next diet and Adam with similar but with jacket potato instead of chips. (He's the health conscious one.)

We were discussing Diana then as seeing her the day before she seemed even more preoccupied than usual; it was difficult to make any kind of conversation, she stuck to Sean's side like her life depended on it.

We went through every scenario but couldn't come up with any ideas. I dismissed him having an affair as he was always working – HOW WRONG WAS I!? Adam had also noticed a change in her, so I wasn't dreaming, as men don't usually notice these things, well Adam doesn't! I had said on the phone to my mum only recently, did she suspect something was wrong, but we couldn't think what. Mum had put it down to the menopause and we were just looking for things that weren't there, but I wasn't convinced of that. I don't know why I didn't ask her what was troubling her, I don't usually hold back but this was different, and when she was ready she would tell us. Diana just could not keep a secret, she was the same when we were children, I'd say don't tell mum and she'd tell her! Looking back I think deep down I knew it would be bad and that I didn't want my bubble to burst. I know it sounds very mean but life was good and I was enjoying my free time. Could I have changed anything? No, I know it would have happened even quicker, his going I mean.

We had left Basingstoke shopping centre listening to the CD in the car as usual; I was feeling happy that Christmas was around the corner. I love Christmas, it is my most favourite time of the year, and I always decorate the house inside and out with lots of bright flashing lights draped round bushes and hanging around our large blossom tree in the front garden. I also have an artificial tree called Douglas Fir Tree. He sings Christmas carols every time you walk near him, he is also decorated with pretty lights, the brighter the better and the more the merrier. Well, over the top I suppose, but that's what I love about Christmas, you can go over the top, it doesn't matter.

I arranged all the different games we played every year; quizzes with silly prizes and picture games and drawing games. I spent literally hours on the Internet looking for quiz questions that fell into every age group. I would go to the pound shop and buy gifts for the prizes. I had wrapped up a German dictionary one year and claimed it was the special fantastic mystery prize knowing full well that everyone would try to win it. Joke on the person that won it!

We would have our Christmas dinners in our own homes, taking in turns; Mum and Dad to me one year then Diana's the next then back to my house for games and tea.

Arriving home from shopping that particular day changed everything. I had phoned my mum to say I had got the package she wanted me to get for her from the health food shop, but my dad answered saying I had better get round to Diana's as Sean had left her. It suddenly all fell in to place.

He walked out on Diana saying he didn't love her anymore, he had been seeing someone twenty years his junior. You can imagine the state poor Diana was in, it broke my heart to see her. She had known for a while but he had been promising that the affair was finished. Diana didn't want us to know as she hoped it would all blow over and save her the embarrassment of telling her family. But they were in constant contact by text, Diana had read many of the messages on his phone, ones sent and received, and unfortunately they both worked at the nightclub where he was a doorman, this is where they first met.

My sister was distraught. To her, her life was over, without him she was lost. How do you comfort someone in a situation like this? And of course the children were so upset and hated seeing their mother so overcome with grief. All I can say is I did my best to comfort her. We talked, hugged, cried together and I tried to reassure her that hopefully he would come back soon, and that more often than not these affairs blow themselves out. (He did come back after nine days but behind Diana's back he still continued to see his girlfriend.)

He heartlessly told Diana he only came back for the sake of the children. He said he would sleep on the settee; and announced he would not stop seeing his girlfriend. Even though Diana's heart was breaking she had no choice but to throw him out. And for the next few years and to this day all our lives have changed.

From the very beginning I had no choice but to take charge of her life. She literally stopped functioning; we were thrown straight into a waking nightmare. He left Diana without any money. I had frozen their joint account at the bank to stop him cashing out any more money. This was recommended by the bank until we could find out why he had taken the money. He had withdrawn all the money from their joint account in two days. He had been having a lot of dental treatment and needed all the money to pay off the bill, but not knowing this we panicked.

We decided to go and see him at his girlfriend's to try and talk things through. Diana hoped he would see sense and come home, or at least agree to sign and unfreeze their account, (it needed both signatures to reactivate it). This was the most important thing as the mortgage had to be paid and bills and food had to be bought and paid for.

I know Diana just wanted to see him regardless of the money, her head was all over the place. At this point I didn't have time to worry about Diana's feelings; money was the priority, without it things were going to be impossible.

He had moved to another town about twelve miles away. So the four of us, me, Diana, Adam and Lauren went to try and speak to him. Lauren said she would knock on the door and ask him to come and speak to them, as we knew he would probably refuse to come out for Diana. He came out as soon as he saw Lauren at the door. I sat in the car waiting with Adam. Diana tried to explain about the account, that she had panicked because he had taken out most of the money. But he refused there and then to sign the form to unfreeze the joint account, and he also told Diana he wasn't going to pay in his wages anymore.

He wasn't interested in what Diana had to say, he looked awkward and shuffled from one foot to the other. I could see he wanted to go. He then coldly told my heart broken sister to get a job. This coming from a guy who never wanted Diana to work! The poor girl had even dressed up a little and carefully applied makeup hoping, I suppose, it would get his attention.

Diana was already in pieces, she was in no state to get a job. He was indifferent to her feelings and walked away while she stood there sobbing. Lauren helped her mum back to the car then we left. The only sound was Diana quietly crying. I couldn't begin to imagine how desolate and lonely she felt at that very moment.

Sean had been the love of Diana's life; she had known him since she was fourteen. They seemed to hit it off right away, and were together from then on.

I know their marriage was different to mine. He worked days as a builder and nights as a doorman; he was hardly at home. I wouldn't have wanted it that way if it had been me but Diana seemed ok with it.

They had a lovely comfy home and two lovely kids, and a fortnight's holiday every year.

They were quite comfortably off with no money worries and a mortgage that would end very soon.

But they never did anything much as a couple. He never took her out for a meal or to the cinema, he just worked. They had the odd trip out on a Sunday mostly to the shopping centre or maybe to visit his family. Behind closed doors were things different? The children seemed perfectly happy being with their mother most of the time. I suppose it was what they had grown up with, kids just accept the way things are; their dad worked a lot, that was it. Sean was home on Sundays but tired because of continuous working day and night, but he did take the kids to the park while Diana cooked dinner. I know he loved his children but unfortunately because he worked most of the time it was always going to cause problems between them.

Men seem to find it easier to walk away from a marriage stupidly believing things will stay the same when they leave. My own first marriage ended after seven years (my choice) because I met Adam but it never once entered my head to leave my children. I know it hit my first husband hard once it came out that I had feelings for someone else. He said he would fight me in court for custody of our children, so I announced I wasn't leaving as I couldn't bear the thought of losing them or being a part-time mum. He could tell I wasn't happy, (even though I tried to act as if everything was ok), and that it wouldn't work between us, so we amicably decided to part, with me taking the children. I suppose I had my cake and was eating it, although for the first six months I suffered terrible guilt taking them away from their father. I never kept them away from him and he had regular access. My children were very young and adapted very quickly. But Liam and Lauren were old enough to feel the hurt and betrayal and chose to blank their father.

Chapter 2

Diana and me

Diana and I were so very different. As children we liked the complete opposite. I loved all sport; she was a typical girlie-girl; hair, makeup, girlie sleepovers, boys, going out. My life was football, tennis, badminton, watching the darts with Dad and the Saturday afternoon wrestling. I liked to go out but I was shy. I did like boys but the shyness was such a burden and so embarrassing for me, I felt safer at home or in a crowd so I could blend in and hopefully not be noticed by the opposite sex. Diana was confident, outgoing and wasn't plagued with shyness like I was; she lit up a room when she walked in, always with a big smile on her face, exuding confidence, with a very infectious, rather naughty giggle.

I didn't take much notice of her relationship with Sean, she never told me much about what they did and where they went and to be honest I wasn't really interested.

All I knew is where he lived and that he smoked and that Diana had started to smoke once she had been going out with him for a while. Mum never liked the idea of us smoking so Diana hid it from her, I didn't let Diana know that I had seen her smoking in our local pub, it was up to her if she told our mum.

They spent a lot of time visiting friends and family, Sean had quite a big family.

I was usually in a sports hall somewhere; there my shyness didn't exist. I excelled in all sport and took to and did well in everything I attempted.

I was two and a half when Diana came along. I wasn't really interested in my new baby sister, her crying annoyed me and she wasn't much fun, until she began to toddle around after me. I remember digging in the garden one day, she bent down to watch me; I had found quite a few worms. After digging in the mud, I laid them on the garden path where they wiggled along. 'What are dem?' Diana asked in her cute baby chat.

'It's mince,' I told her. 'Here, let me put them in your nappy because I haven't got a bag, and then take them into Mum and ask her to cook the mince for our tea.'

Off, she trustingly went while I giggled watching the slimy blighters as they wiggled down her legs as she waddled into the kitchen. She always did as I requested. I wasn't cruel to her and I never hurt her but I found her an amusement with her baby chat and willingness to please her big sister. I remember it as if it were only yesterday and I remember Mum coming out and telling me off although she said it with an amused look in her eyes.

Wherever I went, Diana followed, copying my every move. If I skipped she skipped, if I sang she sang. I was quite independent and was quite happy to play on my own and I preferred to talk to grown-ups, she was like a little shadow always there, following her big sister.

Next door to the left of us they had a gardener and Mum said he would spend ages talking to me and I to him. Mum could see him laughing at the things I would tell him. I could vaguely remember standing at the garden wall enjoying our long chats and his laughing at my childish chatter. I remember the top of his little finger was missing, and that he leant on the top of his garden fork while he listened to my every word. It's strange the things that stay with you. What I talked about I don't remember; only him throwing back his head and laughing out loud.

The next door neighbour on the right of us, a Mrs O'Grady, would also chat to me and Diana over the garden fence. The two of us must have had plenty to say in those days! I know I liked grown-ups and the things they had to say. She once said that Diana was a chip off the old block, (not sure what she meant by that), but the name Chip then stuck. I called her Chip and that's the name I called her from then on.

As we got older we played together more, we would open up Mum's gate leg table and spread a blanket over it and make it our play den. We had cushions, our toys, and Mum would let us picnic under it just like our own little house. We would sometimes play schools and set each other school work, taking turns to be the teacher. Then we would be mums and dads with our dolls. Some days we would spend nearly all day sat in our pretend home. We would also make tents in the garden, weather permitting, and take our pet cat Tammy in with us, much to his disgust as he was whipped up out of his warm slumber and made to be part of our game. He was a fantastically natured pet and a very clever one.

When Tammy wanted to come in at night he would lift up the front door knocker with his paw and let it drop knowing that someone would come to the door to see who was knocking. There sat our daft but very clever cat!

Most of our games were make believe and creative. Mobile phones and computers didn't exist and we didn't spend hours in front of the television as kids do now. There were a few programmes on at about noon but nothing worth watching, well nothing we wanted to watch. There was no morning telly in the '70s and we only had three channels to choose from, so our games were much more important, fun and inventive.

Telly was probably only turned on in the evenings in most homes, daytime very rarely. .

Our first telly was black and white and the picture rolled over and over. You had to give it a sharp thump on the top to stop the bloody picture moving. Thinking about it now it was very funny and also annoying if there was something on you wanted to watch.

Do children have the same imagination now as we did when we were children? Not as much, as television can be on from morning to the evening in the holidays. A shame really but then it isn't safe to let kids have as much freedom as we had then, due to so many unsavoury characters, and there are far more cars on the roads these days, another danger to young children. Most households have computers, computer games, DVD players and most kids have a mobile phone by the time they are ten, I suspect even younger in some families, all the things we would never have owned, because they didn't exist.

Our mother used to say to us, 'Being a child is the best time of your life.' Many a time she would say that when we moaned about something stupid or that we had nothing to do and were bored. But really we weren't bored, I remember always being busy from dawn till dusk.

I look back now after all that has happened and know it was a special time; no cares, no worries, food on the table and a loving family. If I had a wish, it would be to go back to one of those care free days, and warm summers, the days when summer was summer! When the sun shone from dawn till dusk, playing our make believe games, it was safe to play out. We made our way to the woods and climbed trees with our friends, and made camps or played hide and seek amongst the trees; we rode our bikes up and down our streets. We played tennis and rounders, went in for lunch then back out again to continue our play. We didn't need mobile phones then, we came home when we were told, or Else!

I'm glad mobiles hadn't been invented then; so many kids spend their days texting away, it stops a lot of other things being done they don't chat they just text! What would they do with themselves if they were all sent back to the seventies? Would they all hang around phone boxes?

Diana had a wicked sense of humour. We were playing in our back garden one summer evening, the game was a typical '70s game which involved a long piece of elastic sewn together. Two people would stand opposite each other with the elastic stretched about their calves, the third person then had to do various jumps onto the elastic. On this particular day there was only the two of us so the back gate became the second pair of legs, Diana deliberately kept moving while I tried to jump onto the elastic. This made me cross at first then giggle like mad because she wouldn't stop cheating. With all the giggling I was suddenly bursting for the loo. As I was trying to untangle myself from the elastic she let it go 'ping!' and ran into the house shouting back that she too was bursting for the loo and was going first. I followed her in, legs tight together so as not to wet myself and still giggling hoping she would be quick. But she deliberately kept me waiting. I pounded on the door and in her wicked voice she calmly said, 'Yes, can I help you?' Well I laughed even more as she refused to let me in and there in our small hallway outside the bathroom door I peed my pants. My black trousers were soaked and the hall carpet was damp as I couldn't control myself, or the laughing.

I remember our mum wasn't there, I think she was chatting to our next door neighbour, Dad was also out. Finally she opened the door so that I could shower and change, and then clean the hall carpet, all the time she kept on laughing. I begged her not to tell anyone that I had wet myself. 'I might I might not,' she replied. She never did tell anyone. Obviously we had to tell our mother whom also laughed knowing exactly what Diana could be like. (Maybe she was getting me back from the days of worms in her nappy.) It is one time that always stays with me.

As a teenager Diana had quite a few friends and spent most of her time with them. Katie was her best friend, she had fiery red hair, a pretty freckled face and together they were a pain in the neck, to me that is. Don't get me wrong, I liked Katie but when Diana had her to sleep over I never actually got any! Sleep that is, they would incessantly giggle and have farting competitions under the bed covers. At first it was extremely funny, but they didn't know when to stop. It would get to one in the morning and they were still being pains. Mum would come in and warn them that it would be the last time that Katie stayed over, as soon as she left the room there would be peals of laughter from under the covers. In the end I would take a blanket and sleep on our settee in the lounge, and then crawl back in the morning when they were finally fagged out. Of course Katie did continue to sleep over and they continued to be pains.

On one of their dopey escapades they decided to lock Katie in the boot of her mum's car just to see how long Katie could bear the dark confined space.

Unfortunately when Katie was ready to come out Diana couldn't undo the boot. It was then panic stations as Diana had to find Katie's mum and explain where Katie was, and that she was screaming to be let out. They became infamous for their daft and sometimes irresponsible pranks – but that's all they were, just pranks. Nothing terrible, just girls being silly, although if they hadn't got the boot open it would have been a fire brigade job, a time waster that needn't have happened. They were always punished, usually grounded only to be back together within a few days.

The worst thing they ever did was get drunk. Our dad worked for Allied Breweries as a rep and had lots of miniature bottles of drink, which were kept on a drinks trolley in our front room. It was the school holidays. Mum was at work for the morning at the infant school where she was caretaker and I was at the bank where I worked as a cashier. Diana was about fourteen at the time. She invited Katie and another friend round, together they mixed the little miniature bottles and polished off the lot. Never once as children had we ever touched those bottles.

Mum received a phone call from her friend and neighbour saying she was concerned as the TV man (in the seventies you hired televisions if you couldn't afford to buy one and put 50ps in the back to operate them) came to empty the TV (for the rental). He was greeted at our door by my drunk, giggling sister, and her two equally drunk friends. He alerted Mum's friend about his concern for three very inebriated teenagers. Mum immediately returned home, the two friends had scarpered knowing our mother would soon be on her way and didn't want a telling off. Diana, Mum told me later, fell backwards into the bath and bumped her head, luckily she was ok. When I returned from work later that day she was still giggling, burping and she stank of liquor. She wasn't even sick nor did she suffer a hangover which might have taught her a lesson. She was grounded again, this time for a week which never seemed to bother her. After that any drink was locked away.

Diana found school relatively easy, she never seemed to have homework whereas I had loads, she apparently did it on the coach on the way home from school. How that worked I don't know but I was constantly looking in reference books and the encyclopaedias that Mum had bought second hand. I think she just had a marvellous memory and schoolwork came easy to her. I do admit that I took a lot of time from school as my shyness was a real hindrance and anything I couldn't cope with I would practically beg our mother not to send me. She once said that if I had attended more I would have had fantastic grades as they were quite good for the amount of time I took off. My shyness started as I got older and not as the confident young child that chatted to the neighbours. Sometimes I wished I still had that confidence.

Diana loved school and always attended; she was outgoing and wasn't plagued with shyness like me.

She liked fashion, although in the seventies there wasn't really a fashion sense, it was usually jeans and some sort of bright t-shirt and she owned a leather jacket so she thought she looked the bee's knees, and with her long dark thick shiny hair and large green eyes, which she made up with dark green eyeliner, she did! She was the pretty one and I was the attractive one (so I was once told).

I always had my hair shorter, it suited me better. We were both naturally very slim. Oh how I miss my figure now!!

As we got older we spent less time together as I was usually wherever there was some kind of sporting game going on, waiting patiently to be asked to join in. I could hit a ball as hard as any lad my age and I could throw a ball further than a lot of them. Being part of a team or a game helped my shyness; this is when I excelled, which made me popular, and helped improve my confidence.

Diana and I spent more time together when we left our teens behind, especially when I had children, as the one thing Diana adored was kids, anyone's kids; that's how I knew she would make a great mother one day. So when I had John she made a point of visiting me every Thursday on her day off. She loved him and he loved her, she would buy him presents and sweets. She would spoil him rotten, and he loved her to bits.

She was also very generous, especially when it came to letting me borrow her clothes, for the odd works do or a family celebration. My wardrobe was more geared towards looking after kids and playing my sport. Posh frocks were quite scarce in my house, so Diana would let me go through her smart dresses and pretty tops. I would then borrow something appropriate; Diana had quite a lot of smart clothes to choose from. My sister was the most generous person I ever knew. I would then wash, iron and return after use.

When she left school she got a job in a chemist, which was next door to where I worked in the bank. She was a very popular member of staff and liked by the customers as she always had a smile on her face, a great giggler, very friendly and was always willing to look for anything that couldn't be found on the shop shelves. I can honestly say Diana loved her job and was good at it.

She was sent on a few cosmetic courses to learn about the products that they sold. She also did the stock ordering to keep the shop well stocked. Mum always said that when Diana left to have Liam the chemist was never as well stocked as when she had been there.

I usually got home from work before she did as her hours were longer than mine. She'd come in, scoff her tea and then out she went with Sean. I saw my boyfriend a few days a week; the other evenings were spent at the badminton club at the local college sports hall. I loved the feeling you get from smashing a shuttlecock over a net; great way to relieve tension. My brother-in-law Rob calls it smashing a dead budgie over a net. Very funny guy my brother-in-law.

So Diana and I hardly saw each other as we led our different lives. That is, as I said, until I had my children.

Now we had stuff to talk about, as our common bond became children. She had an infectious loud giggle and my children loved spending time with her because she was so full of fun.

And a wicked sense of humour left over from her days with Katie.

Those early days growing up together were carefree, uncomplicated and fun. Our home was comfortable and our mother looked after us very well. We always had a fortnight's holiday every year and we never went without; if our mother could get it she would. I don't mean we were spoilt but we had nice pressies for Christmas and birthdays and when we were old enough to ride bikes she bought us a second hand one each, so we were the same as the other kids in our street that owned bikes. She worked very hard for us both, it's a shame you don't appreciate things until they are far behind you.

Chapter 3

Sean leaving began a series of events that sent Diana spiralling further into deep despair and desperation.

Sean turned up at the house many times mostly to try and see the children. They wanted nothing to do with him, this made him angry and he would bang on the door and windows demanding to be let in; this then frightened them all as he could be quite intimidating. He would shout that it was his house and that he had a right to enter it. We would end up calling the police but he was always gone before they got to the house so in the end we asked the police to visit him and request he stay away as it was upsetting the children. If they wanted to see him they would contact him by phone.

This obviously annoyed him big time as a week or so later, one February evening, Diana had a visit from the police herself. Sean had reported to the police that Diana had attacked him; he also gave the police a list of people who were there at the house with Diana when the supposed attack took place. These included my husband and son James, which is untrue. They were in fact at James's football training in Aldershot and not at Diana's house as he had claimed. This all actually happened on the day after Sean had left for good on 11th December 2007 and not in February, which is when Sean told the police the incident happened.

On the real particular night, 11th December 2007 Sean arrived to collect his belongings, which we had left in black bags on the front drive. As he was pulling away in the car Diana was begging him to stay and pulling at his jumper. She was just so very upset, hurt and angry, she had also kneed him in the privates to stop him entering the house when he had tried to push past her. (In fact I think she let him off very lightly, I would have strung him up by his balls!) I know why he didn't report it until February. It was just tit for tat, he didn't like being told what to do by the police. We had requested to the police that they ask him to leave Diana and the children alone and stop phoning the house or just turning up whenever he felt like it. Even though the police could see by all our statements that we were telling the truth, that nothing had taken place in February, they still had to follow procedure. So on a freezing cold February night we took my shocked trembling and very confused sister at 11 p.m. to the local police station where Diana was put in a cell and questioned, fingerprinted, and then finally cautioned.

We had to take Lauren with us because it was so late; and she was too young to leave on her own, Liam was out with his friends.

As we sat there waiting for Diana, a frightened and confused Lauren sobbed her eyes out for her mother. Through her sobs she stated that she hated her father for doing this to her mum, she was so shocked, as we all were that it had even got to this. It was that very night that Lauren announced that she never wanted to see her father again. My sister was absolutely devastated by her ordeal and this again added to more stress, pushing her further, I'm convinced, towards her illness.

The police even said they wondered why Sean hadn't any scratches on him when they took his statement, but because of rules and procedure they still had to question my sister like a criminal. I don't have a lot of faith in our justice system.

Diana looked so shattered by her ordeal; when she finally appeared at one a.m. in the morning, like a frightened rabbit caught in headlights, her eyes wide and scared from her ordeal. It was so unnecessary to put her through this. She had no money coming in apart from jobseekers allowance; I knew she couldn't take much more and now this to add more salt to the wound.

Diana's thoughts when she went to bed that night must have been how could he do this to her, but she never once said a bad word about him. I feel so sorry for her as looking back she was so hurt and distressed; her life had revolved around Sean and her two children, and now he had gone her world was in tatters.

I was trying my best to keep it all together for them, the three of them were like lost souls. Every letter or bill that arrived Diana gave to me to deal with, her heart was broken and she couldn't cope with anything. Her only thoughts were when would he come home, as time and time again she would ask me if I thought he would come back to her.

She became terrified of every letter that was pushed through her door; she began giving them to me unopened. She just couldn't function, she was a very frightened girl and I didn't know how to pull her out of this situation. I just had to deal with things each day as they presented themselves, my mind was full of my own thoughts and worries. How was I going to get her through this? I knew how much he meant to her. Diana was not going to get over this very easily. How was this going to end, and when would it end? My mind was in constant turmoil and my headache was relentless. Should I speak to him? Could I make a difference? Get them to talk, seek the help from a counsellor, I really didn't know which way to turn. The only time I felt relaxed was once I climbed into bed, although it didn't stop me laying there worrying, as the sister I knew and loved was slowly disappearing in front of me. I actually felt very frightened for her; it was the worst thing to happen to anyone. And Sean may not agree but it was very cruel to leave them in the situation he left them in.

I know his opinion was 'if the children didn't want to see him why should he care,' but situations like this have to be handled so carefully, he should have realised how desperately hurt they were.

Whatever he felt for my sister, the two children should have been considered; they deserved none of this. But unfortunately it is usually the children that end up hurt the most, and it was made worse by their ages, fourteen and seventeen a time when a father and mother are so important. Lauren's schoolwork suffered and Liam refused to work with his father anymore, they both felt so angry towards him. They were both worried about their mum and it was their father and his girlfriend they blamed.

Diana always seemed so strong to me, but it makes you look at your own life and think: could I do things differently? Would Adam leave me one day for a younger thinner person? One thing I know I must do is lose weight. Not because I think Adam may leave me one day, but for my own health; I may get ten years back if I reduce my waistline. I was always thin with a good figure until I was diagnosed with thyroid problems. Then my weight ballooned and here I sit at my computer with my posterior lolloping over the sides of my computer chair (well nearly). The problem with having a thyroid condition makes it tough when it comes to losing weight and my medication doesn't help either, and everything that was happening with Diana was making me turn to comfort eating. I know, excuses excuses, but I had joined Slimmer's World a few years ago, Diana lost an incredible five stone in six months and I only managed a measly nineteen pounds. I didn't cheat but I felt bloody awful as I was always hungry and the weight was taking ages to shift. I was determined to stick with it at all costs, that is until I hit a plateau, the weight just didn't want to shift. At our weekly weigh in, queuing up one fatty behind another, we'd climb on the scales and out loud came, 'Two pound on, Jan. Have you cheated?'

'No I did not.'

'Are you on your monthly?'

'No I am not.'

'Oh you'll probably lose double next week.'

Next week came. 'Only a half pound off I'm afraid, Jan.' It was taking forever to shift my bloody weight although when I received my gold sticker for losing a stone I felt great and really proud of my achievement. I managed a few more pounds then it just stopped; it just wouldn't shift. 'Sod this,' I said to Diana, 'I'm not paying four pounds a week to be told not to shovel food in my mouth, especially when I'm sticking to the diet and nothing is happening.'

So I left. Diana had reached her ideal weight so I wasn't letting her down. And I give her praise, she kept it off for quite a few years. I think when you get older you definitely have to work harder to keep in shape, especially people like me who can look at a piece of chocolate and put on a couple of pounds. Trouble is I didn't only look at it!

So now my routine is totally crap: I'd start a diet every other Monday, then by the Wednesday something would upset me and I'd cheat and then feel angry with myself for ruining my efforts which as you see were not very good. I will admit that one bad night I sat in secret and ate five custard doughnuts. I felt as sick as a pig afterwards and have not done it again since.

All this pressure wasn't helping, and as I said I have been comfort eating, my quick fix for the night! But I'm only fooling myself. It makes you feel good for barely a few seconds. I am the only one that can sort me out and feeling sorry about how I look or feel won't make my weight disappear. I'm not a stupid person. I know if I lose the weight I will feel differently about myself, and I know I will feel healthier just as I did when I played badminton. I was slim, my mood was good and I felt good about myself, and my bloody clothes fitted! All I feel at this present time is embarrassment at my size and self-loathing that I don't have the will power to do something about it.

Chapter 4

At night I selfishly prayed that Sean would come back. It wasn't that I didn't care, but if he came back we all got our lives back. Diana got her life back, I would get back the sister I was missing, and the children got their parents back. The pressure to be the strong one for them all was already starting to close around me. So bang went all diets as the naughty Jan would take over and sneak downstairs and stuff extremely unhealthy food, giving me that brief buzz. I'm a person that likes my own space, and my own company, not all the time, but I'm sure most people like time to themselves. Time to read, do crosswords, pursue hobbies, or listen to music. I had also started writing again; verses for greeting card companies and had sold a few, but with all this happening I had no time to write and be by myself. I am not normally a selfish person but it was a very distressing time. I became snappy with people, and I had to keep it to myself how I was really feeling especially when I was with Diana. I had to be the strong one for her. I know she couldn't help herself and her constant need of my support and reassurance that I wouldn't let her down. Many a time I wished there had been another sister to take a bit of the burden from me and to have someone to phone so that I knew the decisions I was making were the right ones. I didn't like bothering Mum too much as she was worrying constantly about her youngest daughter.

I needed to be there for my niece and nephew who were taking the brunt of the awful situation, day and night, they needed to know I wasn't going anywhere.

Liam had taken his father leaving very badly. Having learning difficulties has made his life hard enough, he is like a fourteen-year-old in a twenty-one-year-old body. He was diagnosed with Dyspraxia when he was at junior school, it causes nervousness, reading, and writing problems along with clumsiness, a short term memory and he finds the concept of money extremely difficult. Without his friends' help when he goes out he would be an easy target for incorrect change etc. It has been impossible to find Liam work that he is able to cope with. I had no choice but to take him to the jobcentre to sign on, luckily there is a disability team who try and help people like Liam find employment but as yet nothing has been found for him. He is now with a company called HF trust (not sure what the HF stands for) and they are in the process of trying to find him a job, where he will get support. I truly hope they will sort it all out for him, it's what my sister would want.

Liam found it very difficult to cope when his father left. He came to see me many a day just to talk everything over. He hated how his mum wasn't coping and how changed she was. She had always been his strength getting him through things that you and I would find easy. I know he wanted things back to how they used to be. I didn't mind him sitting with me and wanting my reassurance as I could see how hurt he was but I couldn't change what had happened for any of them. He is such a gentle loving young man but I really had nothing new to say that could make Liam, Lauren or Diana feel better. All I could do was listen to them while they poured their hearts out; only time could heal their broken hearts. I tried to reassure Liam that he wouldn't always feel like he felt now. But seeing his mother cry continuously upset him even more. I think it helped to have his cousins around him, they gave him strength and seeing his own friends gave him enough distraction to get through his hurt. One person leaving caused a domino effect, I lost my solitude, and choice to do what I liked, and the sister I cared very much for was slowly disappearing day by day. Liam lost the father he had once been very close to. My mother was sick with worry over her daughter. Lauren lost her fun loving mother, and Diana changed from a happy girl to a shell of her former self, clinging to all of us for dear life. Sean's leaving I could do nothing about. I think what I found the hardest was going over it time and time again with Diana every day. She wanted to talk about Sean twenty-four-seven which was draining me mentally, I felt so helpless because I couldn't change the situation for her.

It has been the children's choice not to have contact with their father. Although he has blamed me for driving a wedge between him and them.

That I found very hurtful as all I was doing was being there for them because they needed me to help and support with as much as I could.

Many things occurred that needed sorting out, so as a problem arose I did my best to sort it out. The children were witnessing their mother change day by day. I give them credit; everything that took place they coped with and they are two remarkable children, as they literally had to grow up overnight. They became the adults and tried to help their mother as much as they could.

Diana lived in a lovely spacious house in a much sought after road, with a big garden which was always kept immaculate, now her enthusiasm for it was lost. She was always so house proud. Her large garden was always full of flowers, and her favourite pastime was cooking and hoovering. We jokingly called hoovering her pastime as she did constantly hoover, she liked the place spotless, I even think the cat had the odd suction too. We used to tease her because at one time she actually owned three Hoovers. She was the loveliest caring mum to Liam and Lauren and it was so obvious how much they meant to her. She was a very good cook and made lovely pasta dishes and stir-fries, they were always fed very well. She was a person that liked fun and never minded being teased. She loved clothes; she loved going shopping and she enjoyed her holidays usually to Selsey Bill in Sussex. Her life was pretty simple and easy just how she liked it, she was honest and unassuming with no frills and generous with all things, especially her time, not only for her children but mine also. Because of Liam's learning disabilities she had dedicated her time to get Liam statemented so that he could have the much needed extra help at school.

She attended meetings with his teachers and the Headmaster, writing letters to confirm what she and the school already knew, that Liam had a learning problem.

With much pushing and determination Liam got the help he so desperately needed, a teacher's help to sit with him while he worked, reading and explaining what he didn't understand and at secondary school they provided him with a laptop to do his written work.

Diana also attended many hospital appointments as Liam's consultant was and still is convinced Liam has a syndrome. They will continue to do tests on his blood although they may never find out what caused Liam's problems. He was born prematurely. Diana had an emergency caesarean because she had pre-eclampsia, luckily her midwife had called in to see her and spotted the signs and rushed her in to the hospital. This saved her and Liam's life as the placenta had already stopped working; another day and they both would have been in serious trouble.

Diana was once told by a consultant that had taken up Liam's case that they discover new abnormalities all the time. He is now under Addenbrooke's Hospital in Cambridge. After taking saliva swabs they have determined that Liam and also Lauren have a missing gene. They believe this may contribute to his weight problems and maybe his learning difficulties, although it hasn't affected Lauren in the same way. It will be interesting to see what, if anything they do eventually find.

The hospital has since asked for swabs from their mother and father, this I have not been able to provide for obvious reasons. I notified the hospital straight away.

Diana had lovely neighbours and being a small no through private road everyone knew everyone else. Each taking turns to have the occasional barbecue in the road; celebrating the Queen's Jubilee with a street party.

Diana was very well liked by them all. Easy to talk to and friendly. Game for anything.

But the person I have just described was slowly disappearing and I didn't know what to do or how to bring her back. I kept telling myself and praying that time would heal, or Sean would have a change of heart and come home with his tail between his legs carrying a big bunch of roses. Deep down I knew that was never going to happen.

My days rolled into nights while I sorted out money, taking Diana to appointments, to sign on and then to find a solicitor that offered legal aid, (Sean had already filed for divorce) she was inconsolable when she learned of this. I took her to the doctors as she was getting worse day by day, her speech had become repetitive, and she would slur her words some days, as if she had been drinking. I thought it was the shock of Sean leaving, and that she was on the verge of a breakdown. The doctor I took her to see agreed, as at that time there was no other explanation for her bad speech. He said he would refer Diana for counselling, which would be about a six-week wait.

He started her on anti-depressants to try and help.

Most days Diana came to my house mostly for company and to talk about Sean. Because her speech was becoming bad she repeated the same things over and over again, so my reply was repetitive. As I really didn't know what to say to make her feel better, 'Give it time,' I'd say. 'Let him have his fling then he may come back.' I couldn't say anything negative because it wasn't what she wanted to hear. Secretly I felt he wouldn't return, but I never said that to her, he had left for a women that was twenty-two years younger than him and a different life as she had four young children, he must have felt flattered at her attention in the beginning. Will he ever regret going? I really can't say, we heard many stories about the affair some good some not so good, it was best not to tell Diana as it just pushed her further into depression.

I know rumours go around and stories are glorified all the time as it makes them more exciting to relate. I didn't really care what either of them was doing or feeling, although people were quick enough to tell us what Sean was up too. My main priority was Diana and the children's welfare, and the debt that was increasing day by day and causing Diana so much anguish.

One particular Saturday I took Diana and the children to one of my son's football matches. I invited them all along to get them out of the house, which I often did when Sean was working. We were cheering on the team when Diana suddenly shouted, 'Come on, Yams,' instead of James. We all laughed at her mistake, which even she laughed at.

But nothing entered my head that it was the start of something more sinister rearing its ugly head.

I would have bet my home that it was to do with Sean leaving her and the stress she was feeling. Lauren once asked a doctor did her mother get Motor neurone because of her father leaving. The doctor was honest and said that the stress and unhappiness Diana felt could have triggered it off, and that she may not have had it until she was a much older person. Of course we will never know. It doesn't bear thinking about.

But Diana would still have had Motor neurone at some point. After hearing that, Lauren and Liam do not want anything to do with their father. They have had to cope so long without him in their lives that they got used to him not being around.

I felt so angry about Diana's illness, the Dementia accounted for some of her strange behaviour before she was diagnosed. What was God thinking of; her husband leaving her then making her incurably ill? What had she done so wrong in her life to deserve this? She was so young, and loved her life, and she loved her children more. Some people have charmed lives; others have more than their fair share to cope with. I feel so bitter that she should suffer so, but then you look at world disasters and HIV and others like Diana struck down with these unforgiving diseases that don't give you a bloody chance. They will take you and that's that. I believe your life is already mapped out for you, how you choose to live it is up to you. But you cannot win the battle against Motor neurone or MS or Parkinson's, they have already won. You can change jobs, change partners, change homes but you cannot change your illness the battle is already lost. I'm sorry to sound so pessimistic because there is nothing without hope. Every day I hoped she would live and that a miracle would happen if I prayed hard enough. More and more cancers are cured if you get them early enough but some still become terminal. I hope one day cures can be found, if they are it won't be for a long time and certainly not in my lifetime. I know I sound very cynical but it is the truth, no one beats Motor Neurone, not yet anyway, it doesn't play fair, with cancer you do have hope! Will they one day find the answer to this terrible disease? I know the search will continue until maybe one day they will. I just wish I could have spent a little more time with my sister, and she would have lived long enough to see her children marry, have their own children and watch them grow. That is why I feel so angry because she will miss so much. I get so much fun and pleasure from my own grandchildren, Diana deserved the same.

But I know she will watch them from another safer place, her spirit free from her broken, pain filled body.

I told Liam and Lauren once, 'You cannot see her but she will see you.' I know she will watch them from wherever her spirit is, probably with all the other family members that have gone before her, quite a varied bunch I think, she will definitely be the youngest and the prettiest!

Chapter 5

After eight weeks Diana's appointment still hadn't arrived so on my daughter-in-law's advice I took it upon myself to chase up the appointment. I found the number and rang to find out why we hadn't heard anything. After checking for me, a pleasant lady at the other end of the phone announced that they had nothing about a referral for Diana. I explained about her very bad speech and the awful situation she had been left in, and that she needed help desperately, and that I didn't know which way to turn, to find that help. The lady put me through to a nurse who was very sympathetic and arranged an appointment there and then, and would I accompany Diana to the appointment.

I will be honest, I knew that she couldn't go on her own as her speech by now was very bad, the only things she said clearly were, 'Oh my God,' and, 'Yes I know,' so having a conversation was almost non-existent and I had to get her to write things down, but at times these didn't always make sense. I felt cross at yet another appointment to get to and with no car I was spending money on taxis. I suppose we could have got a bus but I just wanted to get there and get home again. I will admit that about twenty years before I had suffered a nervous breakdown because of an illness. Diana was great then taking my youngest to school and picking up any shopping and even cooking dinners for us. So I had a lot to thank her for as she never got impatient with me but just rallied round and helped me get through my illness. I can honestly say she was a better sister to me than I was to her. I took to my bed from a fear I didn't understand and as I couldn't cope, it was the only place I felt safe. If you've had depression you'll know there is a black hole and all the colours in your life have gone, and the more you try to claw your way out the further you slip back in. There are frightening shadows and irrational thoughts and a fear deep inside that won't be reasoned with, you can't talk yourself out of it, or pull yourself together! It is terror at its worse, at that point you feel being dead is the only option to you. To bring you the peace you so crave. In my case I tried to sleep, as sleep brought respite from the fear of another day to cope with. It is the most frightening and lonely place to be in. I remember once hearing about a woman with two small children who had tried to commit suicide; I remember thinking how could she leave her children? But since experiencing depression for myself it isn't a case of being fed up or down it's a real, serious and terrible feeling. All the good feelings have gone leaving you with a feeling of desperation and hopelessness and that you are slowly sinking into some hollow pit not knowing how to get out and survive. If my husband had not been so patient and supported me I don't know where I might have ended up; in a mental home most probably. My mum recently told me that Diana had told her that she didn't know what to do with me when I was suffering with depression; this made me feel very guilty as not once did she ever show how frustrating and difficult to cope with my illness was. At the time I wouldn't have cared anyway as my every thought was how to survive this. I hope I thanked her for all the help and support she gave me, but I really can't remember the transition from ill to well, it happened so gradually it was all a blur. I don't remember the day I got out of bed and got back to living. But with my fantastic doctor and good medication, and my family's support I came through it. It took a long time before I felt able to cope on my own again. But it does leave you with the fear that it may come back one day. I was experiencing that fear now.

Having to do things that I couldn't control and change I began to worry for myself, as I didn't want to spiral down again. I had usually been able to make my own decisions and if I couldn't cope with some I avoided them. I think people who have experienced any kind of depression will understand where I am coming from, you definitely don't need any kind of stress in your life or as little as possible. I also hate it when people say pull yourself together ('I wish'). It doesn't work like that; being thrown in the deep end you'll definitely drown.

It takes time and patience and medicine, (my lifeline); it made me feel normal again. I'm so lucky Adam was understanding and patient, without that I don't know how I would have ended up. (He was my rock). Diana also. So now I was having to go places and do things that were not my choice, but I did them and made myself go because she needed me, and there was no one to take my place. I had no other options or get out clause. I told myself Diana was there for you so now you be there for her!!

Some days the frustration I felt with Diana was bad. I have never been very patient so I wanted everything done yesterday. I wanted her diagnosed and made better so I could go on with my life. And I wanted her happy again. But I never once showed how I felt some days. I hope she knows that I always loved her and that my waking thoughts were of her, and again before I shut my eyes at night I'd say a prayer for her. I just felt powerless to make her happy again. I enjoyed my time with Adam and at fifty I think you have earned that time, your children growing up gives you the reward of more time to spend with each other.

Now that was practically gone Adam and I would sometimes sneak off, just to get away from the constant phone calls from doctors, solicitors, nurses, counsellors, benefit people and the never ending visits to various appointments etc. That's when we visited the Little Chef open until ten p.m. It was a place to go and unwind, drink tea and coffee or in my case stuff my face as stress turned me to food.

We would discuss everything that was happening, when would it be over? Why couldn't Diana snap out of this low mood and talk again? Couldn't she accept he wasn't coming back and that he wasn't worth all her heartache? I understood her low mood but in her case anti-depressants wouldn't make him return to her. I knew it would take time her getting over him but I wished it would be soon, I wanted her to be the happy smiling sister I was missing. My friend and shopping partner had gone.

Was it fair to have a holiday that Adam and I had booked earlier in the year with all this going on? It felt wrong to laugh and enjoy things that gave her no pleasure. We would also ride around in our car and listen to CDs singing along. These few things did recharge my batteries enough to face the next day.

I also have a few good friends that I see and I thank them for letting me moan and share the problems that were in my thoughts every waking minute.

I must have been the most miserable company during those days. Even my poor dogs got moaned at; muddy paws, too many dog hairs; things that never bothered me before got blown out of proportion.

I've realised that situations you are in, especially what Diana was going through, don't just go away. You just have to deal with them, face them head on. I would tell myself everything was solvable, wasn't it? So no amount of wishing or feeling sorry for myself would alter the situation I was in. I had to tell myself constantly that Diana needed me. I remembered that when I had needed help and support she was there for me. I know now the frustration she must have felt with me but she never showed it.

I cried many times as the pressure got worse, the endless phone calls I made to get account numbers changed for her, and visits to the bank as Diana had to have her own bank account since Sean wouldn't unfreeze the joint one. It was extremely difficult when phoning companies to explain the situation Diana had been left in and then to be told they could only speak to the bill payer, I would then explain the bill payer had left and his wife, my sister, was unwell and that it was me they spoke to if they wanted the bills paid. Some were sympathetic, some said they needed some kind of proof before they could change bank details etc. All I know is your life is run by letters, bits of paper, reference numbers, codes, computers and passwords and if you're dealing with someone else's life you are fu-----ked. Luckily I was already an appointee for Diana's income support which saved so much hassle when she finally became too ill to even give her permission for me to speak. The form filling was the biggest bugbear and time consuming. I had to type endless letters to various utility companies then get Diana to sign them. I cancelled direct debits she couldn't afford, and ones she didn't need. I had to plead with her building society to hold off the mortgage repayments as the only money coming in was £50.95 a week. This apparently is what the government says we can live off. Well I'd like David Cameron to live on it, pay bills and feed himself. Diana's child benefit was increased which helped a little and because her ex was not paying a penny I contacted the CSA to make him pay something which was a pittance and took ages before any payments came through. In fact our mother for a year paid for their food every week – £60 including food for the cat.

Without her help they wouldn't have eaten.

But at the end of the day it is all in the past (although I will never forget what they went through). We survived through sheer determination and with the financial support of our mother (the bit of pension she had saved). I don't know where all this would have ended up or rather where they would have ended up! Our mother was a brick; without her support things would have become impossible, and thank you to my friend Jenny. She knows why I am thanking her, my best friend of thirty years and one of the best people I know.

We made endless visits to Diana's solicitor, usually by taxi as all these trips were so time consuming. Extravagant I know but I didn't have time to spend waiting for buses and looking after a sick sister. And running two homes was definitely affecting me, so a taxi got us there and back quicker than a bus. Either I paid the fare or Mum paid the fare or we used her free counters that pensioners received from the council. It's a shame that they changed those to bus passes, which my Mum and Dad will never use as they are too frail to catch a bus let alone walk to the bus stop. A taxi came to the house – much more sensible – whoever changed the system didn't consider the elderly who aren't good on their legs. So my parents will never use their bus passes.

I could probably ring and complain to the council on their behalf as if I believe something is wrong or a cause needs fighting then I don't usually leave it, but I really didn't have time to take on the council as well. Maybe soon, who knows!

Mum would sometimes come with us to keep us company which I liked as Diana couldn't say much. I think Diana liked it when Mum came as she was extra company and it was someone for me to chat to while Diana listened in.

Every day there were endless letters to type and thank goodness my son James taught me how to do attachments on the computer which has been a godsend in sending information to various people, companies, and Diana's solicitor. Also sending requests for all her endless amounts of medication by email to the doctors saved me a trip to the surgery, as eventually she would be taking a lot for her illness.

In April 2008 Diana finally saw a counsellor called Ellen; I explained everything that had happened. I then stayed downstairs while Diana was taken upstairs and introduced to Ellen's colleague also called Diana. I don't know what was said but one thing they told her to do was to try and sing at home, they were hoping this may help get her vocal chords working properly again.

On one of Diana's weekly visits I was called into a session as Ellen was finding it difficult to get anything from Diana or even understand her. I am very tearful now as I now know that it hadn't mattered how hard Diana had practiced or sung, her voice would never have come back. I can see her now sat there, her forlorn sad face looking down to the floor, obviously very embarrassed, her hands clasped together in her lap twiddling her thumbs round and round, and myself and Ellen saying just try a little harder but all she could say was, 'Yes I know.'

I probably sounded impatient and eager to leave. If I could turn back time now I would hug her and say, 'Don't worry, Diana, you did good today. Let's go home now,' but I didn't. I had convinced myself it was all about missing Sean and that's what I stuck to until I knew different.

One thing all this has taught me is to try and be a little more patient. I went to quite a few sessions with her waiting downstairs in the waiting room; I never knew what Ellen said to Diana during the rest of these sessions.

She would come out sometimes smiling, other times very upset. I suppose it was her frustration as like me she was waiting for a miracle to happen, all we wanted was her voice back and her well again and the old Diana to reappear. I didn't know then it was never going to happen.

Chapter 6

But things took a different turn and Diana's problems took a back seat for a while. Our mother had been feeling unwell and had made a few trips to the doctor. She had been suffering from many bouts of cystitis and in one urine sample the hospital had found blood in her urine. Immediately she was referred to the Urology Department at the Royal Berkshire Hospital, where using a long tube with a camera the doctor found a cancerous lump in her bladder. I can tell you that knocked me and Mum for six. I always thought my mum was indestructible, now we had another battle on our hands. All these trips to so many appointments with Diana were already wearing me out, and now my mum had cancer. I hate that word it meant awful things could happen.

A week later Mum and I sat together in the consultant's room, we were told that the cancer was confined to her bladder and that because of her age they were reluctant to remove it (the bladder) as it was a very big operation especially for someone Mum's age. We were told that she may not survive such a big operation as it was a traumatic thing to get over. One choice they recommended to my mother was a wash, which is what doctors used to treat TB years ago. The consultant said that it was good at stopping cancerous cells growing. I felt slightly lifted, as I know my mum and I both feared the worst. She had to come in every week on a Monday for six weeks and have the wash inserted into her bladder then after three months they would check her bladder again. As we walked away we both felt a bit better although neither of us discussed the future or the outcome. I find it hard to talk about it especially to my mum. I tend to make jokes and make people laugh; I take after my dad in that way. It's how I deal with difficult situations. It's almost like if you don't mention it, it won't happen. So that's why I skipped around the subject. I hated the idea of my mum worrying about it as the constant worry over Diana was hard for her to cope with, and now the bloody C word. Of course having cancer was no joke; it wasn't going away on its own and had to be dealt with for as long as it took.

And deal with it we did.

Mum started her treatments a week later; early every Monday morning we went to the urology dept where a nurse called Becky inserted the washes. Mum then had to keep it in her bladder for two hours. The stuff must have been pretty strong because she was told to put bleach on top of it before she flushed the loo after her first wee. Imagine the headlines: woman blows up Berkshire with contaminated urine!!

We could then go straight home, so providing we had booked the first appointment (I did a block booking) we were in and out pretty quick.

The next day she felt pretty sore and had to keep drinking to wash the stuff through. When we got home she went straight to bed as her bladder felt sore and it stung when she had her next wee. After the third day she felt almost back to normal.

Life continued on as before; over to spend time with Diana, sort out any problems, and deal with any post, spend time with Liam and Lauren as life was pretty sombre for them. Then Diana back over to me for company. I also helped with Lauren's homework; maths being her weakest subject, unfortunately mine also. Attend hospital treatments with Mum, attend appointments with Diana, run my own home, feed the family, feed the dogs, meet myself coming backwards!

One day rolled into the next, Easter had been and gone. To be honest I don't even remember it, apart from the usual exchanging of the eggs and a tea at my house; quite uneventful really.

Adam and I managed to have a week's holiday in June, which I had booked the year before. I was convinced that we would have to cancel as I kept waiting for the next crisis to rear its head.

But we got to Sennen Cove in Cornwall as planned. We stayed at a lovely little house on the seafront, it had a huge front room window; our view was superb. The little shelves dotted about the rooms had ornaments to do with the seaside, like the wooden seagull in the window and the little china lighthouse on the bookshelves, and the harbour picture on the wall. All the things I would have on display if I had been fortunate enough to own a beautiful little place like this. The most noticeable thing was the salty smell of the sea and the freshness it brought with it, the kind of freshness that clears your head. It's times like these you cannot believe there are so many problems in your life. Yellow Sands Cottage took us away from all that; for one week we left the problems behind us. I just relaxed and read and relaxed and took daft photos; but that's another story, nothing naughty just silly! (My ridiculous sense of humour!) Of course I wondered how everyone was; my thoughts always went back to home. I felt so guilty going and leaving everyone behind, so I sent postcards home nearly every day writing silly things about me scuba diving then shark fishing and pot holing, and rock climbing, then Adam and I jogging every day. Well anyone that knows me, knows that was the last thing we would do, maybe believable when I was younger and slimmer. To those at home it would be comical. I even sent postcards that were funny and not of sea views as I didn't want Diana and the kids to feel sad at not being on holiday.

The week went incredibly quickly, just as our life was at present, zooming by, our days were pretty full exploring the Cornish coastline and stopping for many cups of tea; some of these with a good old Cornish cream tea – lovely! We visited Lands End, and the Eden project; we were very impressed with the plants and flowers and the two domes and the incredible metal man made of all household appliances – a very clever piece of artwork and a must see for people visiting Cornwall.

I love places like Mevagissey with its many trinket shops, galleries and little fisherman cottages and the narrow winding streets all leading to the harbour. Then Padstow; again a favourite with many Rick Stein fans, now more famous because of his association and probably even busier because of it, but I liked its charm and hustle and bustle, then there are the quieter places like Charlestown and Porthleven.

But my most favourite time is relaxing in a deckchair overlooking the sea, with my nose in a book, letting it fall now and again to gaze at the beautiful view, the sun shining across the water, glistening with every rise and fall of the waves. Everyone deserves this, I remember thinking; peace, warmth, relaxation, happiness, contentment. Especially my sister and the children.

My most favourite place is Treyarnon Bay, I like sitting above the beach on the cliffs. There is a Y.M.C.A and café where you can get delicious rolls and baguettes. My favourite is a tuna roll with a cup of refreshing tea, or a cold coke depending on what you fancy, and the loos are not far as after three kids I can sometimes pee for England. I recommend anyone visiting Cornwall that they pay Treyarnon Bay a visit. Not all at once please as I like a bit of space on the cliffs!

Across the bay on the opposite cliffs are a few, and probably, no definitely, very expensive large houses. I don't know if they are lived in all year or holiday lets but how often do I dream that I have won the lottery and gone with a wad of notes offering to purchase one of these most exclusive homes? Eh, then I wake up.

They are probably priceless as I know I wouldn't be tempted to any amount of money if I owned one, please God!

But no sooner had we unpacked; it was time to pack up again. I felt very sad this time leaving Cornwall and Yellow Sands Cottage and its beautiful sea views.

It was so much harder this time leaving knowing there was so much taking place at home. To be honest I felt anxious about going home as trying to get Diana well again was taking its toll on me.

As soon as we returned there were problems that needed sorting, bills to pay, with very little money. The cat needed to go to the vets because she had a lump, it luckily was nothing serious. There were letters and appointments to sort out and Diana still looked so very sad, her speech no better.

I think she felt relieved when we returned home, safer somehow and company again for her and the children.

Adam and I took them out whenever we could to try and cheer Diana up and give them a day away from the same four walls. We went to Southsea one day. Knowing how I feel when I'm near the sea I thought it would lift her spirits, we had a bite to eat in a little seafront café called Rocksbys. The staff are really friendly and were used to seeing Adam and I on the odd Sunday we managed to get away.

After we had eaten (Diana was already beginning to struggle with food, we had no idea what was around the corner) we went along the seafront to the little indoor market. I love looking around as it sells all sorts of reasonably priced things; my favourite is the bookstall. The books are reasonably priced and have every different genre; I had bought quite a few in recent times. We bought some sweets then went next door to the arcade where I like to play the bingo machine. Lauren enjoyed this as well. I had given Diana a cup full of 2ps to play on the slot machine. As I watched her she just shoved in one 2p after the other until they had gone, she didn't wait for the arm to move backwards and forwards like you normally would it was like she was just thoroughly bored, in another world almost, going through the motions. It is so difficult to explain but by the end of the day she seemed like she was on another planet, her disinterest seemed even worse. I took it that she didn't really want to be there, that a day out to the seaside was not enough to lift her spirits a little bit. I thought then that her heart must be well and truly broken and that she would never get over losing Sean. But of course I now know that it was the Dementia affecting her strange behaviour. I have no idea what she could have been feeling or thinking as she stood there automatically shoving the 2ps into the machine. I don't understand her type of Dementia that well.

On another occasion we went to the zoo. She actually seemed quite bright that day, smiling, enjoying the warm day. Looking back at the photos we had taken she looked really well so to me it was like a small breakthrough. She liked the animals and pointed to them like a child would. It was a very hot day so it was nice to find some shade later, all of us enjoying an ice cream which Diana made a complete mess of but thoroughly enjoyed! We set off to Porchester Castle which is by the sea and about six miles from Portsmouth. We sat in the shade again, as the sun that day was far too hot to sit in. We watched the many boats that sailed by, I remember thinking how I wished I had been in one of those boats and that we were all as happy as the people sailing by, a normal happy family doing normal fun things.

We chatted away to Diana; she just nodded and smiled and said, 'Yes I know,' when appropriate. I remember glancing at her from time to time. She looked the most relaxed I had seen her in a long time, sat on the grass looking out to sea a half smile on her face. I felt quite happy when we dropped them off later on that evening.

'She did seem to enjoy it today, Adam, didn't she?' I asked.

'I think so she seems better away from home'.

I liked to see her smile and relax and that's how she seemed that day. I hoped it was an about turn. And it definitely did Lauren good to get away for the day.

Mum's time to visit hospital again came very quickly and as I said before, the weeks just rolled into themselves, and the days seemed like a hazy blur. Mum was due to stay a few days in hospital while they checked her bladder. Unfortunately it was not good news; the cancer cells had returned so the surgeon removed them. Mum stayed in a bit longer to recover. I must admit those washes are bloody good! Not.

I'm sure they do work on some patients but Mum wasn't the lucky one.

It took her a bit longer to recover this time but she was to have a little break from the next lot of washes, which I think she was relieved to be having. For her age she was coping very well. I believe that it was the constant worry of Diana that took the focus away from herself.

Chapter 7

One day I was looking forward to which was fast approaching was my oldest son John's wedding on 30th August. I had tried to lose a bit of weight, which should have been a lot of weight, but every bad day, and there were many, I just sat and comfort ate, telling myself, 'I'll start again tomorrow.'

Funny that, because tomorrow never came. I had sent for hundreds of pounds worth of clothes hoping the next outfit would be the one, only to bag it up and send it back. Being so overweight my boobs are gargantuan beasts, I can't believe women like to go bigger! I was trying to find an outfit that hid them. Then I had to find a pair of suitable and comfortable shoes; the handbag funnily enough wasn't a problem.

The wedding day was fantastic, we couldn't have asked for better weather. Chloe my new daughter-in-law looked beautiful in her wedding dress, and my three sons and Chloe's brother looked very handsome in their very posh suits with matching lilac waistcoats and ties. The four bridesmaids looked amazing, their hair had been expertly done by Chloe's mum, the colours of their dresses were beautiful shades of lilac and purple; these colours were the theme of the wedding.

The hall was decorated with the same colours; the balloons were lilacs and purples with matching ribbons and although the tablecloths were all white the accessories were again in the same colours. I must admit the hall had been completely transformed – I should know I had helped get it ready along with Chloe's brother Geoff and Mark my middle son and his girlfriend Kylie. Because of John's big passion for football the tables were named after famous footballers. The cake which was beautiful was black and white because he supports Newcastle F.C. I hope he appreciates how easy going Chloe is, not many brides would agree to a black and white wedding cake! But it did look amazing!

Chloe's sister-in-law and also one of her bridesmaids Anna had made the cake and funnily enough Anna's granddad back in 1978 had made my wedding cake, a very small world we live in!

Obviously she got her talent for cake making from her granddad.

The wedding itself was lovely and videoed by Adam. The speeches were hilarious but unfortunately because his arm ached from holding the camera so long Adam rested his arm then and forgot to video the speeches, much to John's dismay when he found out. He was really upset as they were the best bit, but it wasn't really Adam's fault. Any of us could have reminded him but we were so engrossed in the hilarity of the extremely funny speeches. John still brings it up now and again to try and make Adam feel guilty. It works!

The food was simple but very tasty; an assortment of cold meats, pastas, and salads with strawberry gateaux to follow. It was delicious; champagne for the toasts and various wines on each table.

My mum who was in between her next lot of washes looked frail, she said she felt ok, and was thoroughly enjoying the whole occasion. It was an incredibly hot day which was very lucky as most of August had been very wet; so many photos were taken with beautiful blue skies in the background, the most perfect of days!

The photographer was a friend of Chloe's who was studying Photography at college so it was a bit cheaper for John and Chloe and gave her friend some experience of being a wedding photographer. Chloe completely trusted her as she had attended Photography college for a year already.

I didn't find out until later that week that Diana had been crying for Sean while waiting for Adam to pick them up for the wedding. I know she must have felt terrible without him at her side, but she seemed to enjoy the day so I hadn't given it a thought as to how she might be feeling. I suppose I should have realised but being so busy and helping with the preparations I got lost in the moment. I thought she was ok as she danced a lot with me and Lauren at the evening's disco.

Her speech was very bad that day, as she struggled to make herself understood. Luckily people knew how she was so they didn't try to make her speak or try to chat to her, and she stuck by my side like glue which sometimes annoyed me. Thinking back it was the only thing she could do as she didn't want to be put in an awkward situation where someone unaware of her condition tried to start a conversation with her. There is so much I look back at now and wish I could change but at the time I didn't think as I was so caught up in the excitement of the day, and I didn't know how incredibly ill she was becoming. I was just enjoying myself dancing and mingling with various friends. I actually thought that Diana had enjoyed herself with the dancing and the whole occasion but she just went home and continued drinking and cried herself to sleep. She must have felt so lonely and confused. Thinking back I know there was no more that I could have done to make her situation different. Her illness, although we didn't know it, was already taking a firm hold and it would take a long time until the diagnosis came.

I knew she had been drinking in the evenings, probably to blur her feelings but it was worrying Liam and Lauren, so I went with Mum to see her and said that drinking wouldn't bring Sean back, that if she continued I wouldn't help her (cruel I know but it was getting worse). She had a cry and I knew I would have to keep an even closer eye on her. But I did reassure her I would never desert her. The two children must have found it so hard to cope with the way their mother had become, I can only imagine what they witnessed when Mum and I were away from the house, her constant tears and deep despair far worse than we ever saw. They never complained much, as their love and loyalty to Diana was remarkable. It was such a sad time for them both trying to accept all that was taking place. I know deep in my heart that none of us could have done any more than we were doing – it wasn't humanly possible, especially with so much going on.

Chapter 8

September came and went then October. Adam had been complaining of feeling unwell. He had been to visit his Mum in Lyme Regis and he phoned me to say that he had felt unwell again especially after climbing the steep hill that leads to his sister Sarah's house. I told him that he was going to the doctors the next day and no arguments.

For a while now Adam had been complaining of a strange feeling in his throat and mouth especially after he had eaten. I could only think of indigestion but to be honest, with my days being so busy with Diana it wasn't that I ignored Adam, but if he had complained of pain in his arms it would have rung alarm bells. Adam always ate so quickly that I just told him to eat slower and if it wasn't any better he should make an appointment to see his doctor. But as usual it's always the wife that takes control and after the Lyme Regis episode I made the appointment and made him go. What makes me cross now is that when Adam had visited his doctor he was sent to the nurses' station to be wired up to a heart monitor, but what the nurse didn't do was shave his incredibly hairy chest, believe me he could have doubled up for King Kong.

If she had shaved his chest, and attached the wires to his skin it might have prevented what happened two days later. (That was what the ambulance man told Adam.) The reading hadn't shown anything suspicious and he came home saying he was fine but that he would receive an appointment within the next week to go on the treadmill at the Royal Berkshire Hospital.

I remember the evening like it was five minutes ago. Adam came in from work with the usual, 'What's for dinner, girl?' and as soon as he had eaten the same happened again; the weird feeling in his throat but this time his complexion was really grey. I was flummoxed as to why indigestion would make him feel so ill, so I rang our son James and asked that he get some Gaviscon and could he get it now. I had told Adam there were some Rennies by our bed, as he got to the top of the stairs I heard aloud groan then a thump where he fell to his knees. I just knew deep down what it was, and without even thinking I phoned 999. I could hear Adam saying God it hurts. All the time the lady on the end of the phone kept telling me to keep calm and that the ambulance was on its way, she instructed me to turn on any outside lights, which we don't have, and look out for the ambulance. I did as she said, whilst all the time she spoke to me. Luckily I didn't go up to Adam as the ambulance had pulled up half way down my road at the wrong house, so as I looked out I waved until they spotted me, they were there within seconds. As they turned up so did James. I don't know why but I felt so calm as the men rushed past me; relief I suppose because they were there, and disbelief that this was actually happening. I followed them up stairs, they had sat Adam on the bed; he looked awful and even greyer than before. They asked if he drank or smoked and his age. 'I don't think it's anything too bad,' said one, 'but we will check him out in the ambulance.' Fifteen minutes later one ambulance man came to the door, by then I was pacing up and down the hallway.

'I'm afraid we are picking something up on the heart monitor. He's ok, we've given him some medication, just get some bits together and follow us to casualty.'

I felt my legs buckle beneath me, I managed to pull myself together and grabbed whatever I could lay my hands on. By now my other two sons had arrived. I continued to shake with nerves in the car, all the time saying to myself don't let him die please God don't let him die! What I found out later was that the ambulance man had correctly shaved Adam's chest. They told him that the nurse should have done the same because the sticky pads would have only stuck to his hairs and not given a proper reading because they weren't touching his skin. I'm not a doctor and the nurses at the surgery will probably say that they did everything correctly, but would it have made a difference between Adam having a heart attack and not having one? Would it have shown something earlier if the nurse had shaved his chest?

I knew when we got to the hospital what they would say but it didn't hit me until a doctor said it. 'He's had a heart attack, you can see him but only one person at a time please.' My legs turned to jelly again, this couldn't be happening not my Adam, he was never ill. I was the one that got things and had depression and had half my thyroid out and had various women's problems and carried too much weight, why wasn't it me lying there?

I had made Adam go to the doctors two years previously due to high cholesterol in his family. It was high but he was told to watch his diet, drink Benecol drinks and use Benecol butter. One of the ambulance men said they wished doctors didn't advise people to switch to these products, as Adam would have needed to drink a vat of the stuff every day to bring down his cholesterol. I personally think doctors need to make it very clear how serious high cholesterol is to scare people like Adam into doing something to change how they eat and exercise. I could have been a lot stricter with his diet and encouraged that he exercised. I don't know if it would have been enough to prevent what happened, but it might have. Sometimes medicine is the only way to go but it wasn't offered to him originally.

As I walked through the curtain I didn't know what to expect. He actually looked better than two hours previously, his colour was so much better, the greyness now gone from his face, he had wires sticking out from everywhere and the sound of his heart beating filled the cubicle. It sounded ok to me, and thank God it was beating! Poor thing, he looked so scared and was trying to be brave, I on the other hand felt like collapsing to the floor. Almost like if I touched him he would break. We weren't allowed to stay long but I could phone when I wanted to through the night to check how he was.

I felt so anxious but I couldn't cry. I think it was the shock and disbelief. I was in a sort of daze while I tried to think why our family was being punished and there wasn't a thing I could have done to prevent it. All thoughts of my sister had left my head. I now had a sick husband to look after and I still didn't know how serious it was as a doctor would see him the next morning. So that night I phoned quite a few times, I had to, I couldn't sleep and I certainly couldn't relax. A nurse told me they had hooked up a telly for him because he was finding it difficult to sleep or cope with what had happened. Adam had requested a T.V. to try and take his mind off his heart attack. I also phoned his work colleague Paul even though it was late I knew he wouldn't mind. He took it hard as Adam never took sick days, he never caught colds and I've never known anything that kept him off work until now.

As I lay in our bed I shook with worry; I tossed and turned, I tried to watch telly as well but I couldn't hear what they were saying. I prayed to God not to take him from me as he had always been my rock, he supported me when I couldn't cope with things and situations because of my depression, he was great company and I loved him loads so I prayed as hard as I could hoping that there was a God and that he would hear me and that all we were going through was just a nasty dream! Pinch! No it was real so deal with it, Jan.

The next morning my middle son Mark, turned up to keep me company. I wasn't allowed in to see Adam until two o'clock as the visiting times are very strict in the ICU, so the morning dragged slowly. Diana appeared at my door when she knew what had happened to Adam and I'm so sorry to say that I couldn't cope with her that day. I feel so cruel now but all she could say to me was, 'Oh, my God.' If I had taken time to look at her I would have seen how sorry she was for me, the tears are streaming down my eyes now, because she had come to see me because she cared about me. I knew she couldn't talk to get over how she felt, but I was distracted and didn't want to chat to her, my mind was thinking of Adam and what the outcome was. I feel so cross with myself as her life for those two and a half years were so incredibly sad. Could I have done more? Sitting here now I could have hugged her and thanked her for her concern and told her that we were off soon, but I didn't. I was finding it very hard to deal with the fact that she couldn't talk and that the conversation was always one sided. I actually felt strange being around this Diana, I just didn't know her, I wanted my old Diana back, she would have been great in this situation. My God how must she have felt; she couldn't even tell us what she was thinking, she must have been so scared. I am so sorry, Diana and I thank you now for coming to see me, and for being there for me when you knew about Adam. But in all honesty I didn't know how ill you really were. I'm not a very tactile person and I have had to learn to be more patient, but mine was being tested to the limit.

I now had three people to think and worry about. It was a real bad nightmare, the difference was, I was really living it!

I did however keep trying to reassure Diana that once she got over her ex and by seeing her counsellor frequently she would soon recover. Many times I had to think of things to say so she could say, 'Yes I know,' or just nod or shake her head. This sometimes proved very difficult and quite draining.

I can honestly say that I didn't know this Diana. I didn't know how to be with her and to be honest the way she had become frightened me, because I didn't know how to deal with it.

Mark and I got to the hospital and down to ICU just before two p.m. You cannot enter until they turn on the lights in the corridor, which indicates visitors are allowed to enter. The first thing I saw was Adam sat up in bed with a big grin on his face. His skin looked a funny colour, a sort of orangey yellow. He announced, 'It's all been done.'

'What do you mean "done"?' I asked.

'The doctors have inserted a stent,' he told us. The yellowing on his skin was anaesthetic wash. I didn't believe him at first, it just seemed too straight forward. Too easy almost.

'I had a blocked artery, and they fixed it by inserting a stent.'

He showed me a drawing which showed where they had placed the stent and that the blood was flowing through nicely. There was another part of his heart on the left which had slight furring. The doctor was considering putting another stent in.

As we talked his Irish doctor came to see him so I took my chance to ask if he would be inserting a stent on his left side.

'Maybe, maybe not,' he said in a strong Irish accent. 'I think everything looks fine the blood is getting through nicely.' I kept asking him questions.

'Is it ok to leave the left side, and won't it cause another attack?'

He replied that the heart was clever and the blood was finding its own route round. 'I think it will be fine and don't worry.' With that he was gone.

I couldn't believe how easy and matter of fact he had made it seem, like he had removed an annoying splinter not performed heart surgery. If it had been one of his main arteries Adam would have been transferred to London to have a bypass operation, so he had been extremely lucky.

Adam stayed in hospital for four days, incredible! I felt very nervous about bringing him home. Mark took me in to collect Adam. On our journey home whilst in the car Adam was very quiet, and kept bouncing his legs up and down, I knew that was a nervous thing. 'Are you ok?' I asked him.

'Yes,' he snapped back, 'I'm fine just don't ask.'

This wasn't like Adam to snap, I had to go very carefully and not keep on although it's difficult when you are worried. When we got home he would only sit at the dining room table, he didn't want tea or anything to eat. The dogs were pleased to see him and over excited but he didn't want them jumping up. I knew he was finding it difficult being away from the security he felt being in the hospital, so I suggested that we played cards. I had to take his mind off himself and concentrating on something else. After an hour I was becoming bored playing rummy, I had dinner to cook and dogs to feed and then take out, I racked my brain as to what he could do to take his mind off himself, then it hit me, he had liked playing the boys hand held Tetris game, something they had as a present one Christmas – that would give him something to focus on. Luckily I remembered coming across it whilst looking for something else in the cupboard. I found some new batteries and good it still worked and believe me it was a Godsend.

When he didn't play that we played cards, if not he watched the history channel on Sky. All the time I kept him occupied so he didn't have time to worry about his health.

Thank goodness for Sky telly as I also encouraged him to watch documentaries as he loves anything to do with history, especially the first and second world wars.

Luckily he always slept well at night so he didn't lay in bed worrying about himself, it was me that was doing the worrying. I prayed hard, make the old Diana come back I missed her, make Adam recover completely and make my Mum's cancer go. It wasn't asking much was it? Was anyone listening? I doubted it but I would keep praying regardless.

After a week Adam had to start a little exercise, walking a little further each day. One day we were allowed as far as the shops so we decided to walk there and on the way back call into my Mum's for a cup of tea then finish the journey, but I could tell as soon as we started shopping Adam was getting agitated.

'You don't like it in here do you?' I asked.

'No can we hurry up please?'

He told me that he suddenly felt panicky being away from the house, we had his phone and his heart spray with us but he felt uncomfortable being around so many people again.

After that the walks we took were never very far from the house. Just across the road from our house was a park so we walked around a little further each day, once round, twice round increasing the amount each time, so he still got his exercise but could see the house where he felt safest. After two weeks he said he felt well enough to walk a little further so we called into some friends and had tea and a chat, but on the way home I noticed straight away he was quiet again. By the time we were indoors he was panicking, pacing up and down and breathing deeply. Mark, my middle son had called round and said I should phone an ambulance just to be on the safe side. I really thought Adam was having another heart attack, please God no I thought. He was checked over, his heart was beating a little fast but to be safe they said it was best to be checked over in the hospital, so we ended up in casualty again, Adam wired up again, blood taken, blood pressure, the works. After what seemed ages the doctor came in with the blood results, he told us that everything was fine and that Adam's heart was beating faster than normal because he had panicked. I knew then that we had done too much that day and that Adam wasn't ready to visit friends yet, so again we kept near to our home and I let him do what he felt he could cope with, he liked the attention he was getting from visitors, he felt safer in his own home and the phone rang every day; if he was tired I spoke if he felt ok he would talk. Although I had found out that on his second day in hospital he had phoned his work to check on his month's figures. His boss had told him that he shouldn't even be thinking of work and to concentrate on getting better. His boss Kevin also rang me to tell me that Adam had rung and to tell him not to even think of work until he was fit. I was livid. It didn't actually surprise me as Adam constantly worried about sales figures etc., so I had to have a sharp word with him. He was more important than work and if he didn't forget about work I would unplug the phone and hide it if he didn't rest and do as he was told. My threat actually made him laugh as he knew I would carry it out if he didn't behave himself.

'Don't mess with the wife,' he said.

'Too true,' I replied.

Slowly and in the right direction Adam began to realise he was ok. The ambulance man had told him that many heart attack victims end up back in hospital because the realisation suddenly hits them and panic and fear take over and the patient ends up in hospital really for reassurance that they are ok. I know it must be the most frightening thing ever.

After four weeks he was allowed to drive again, he also started keep fit classes every Tuesday and Thursday morning. These were for heart attack patients. A guy from the hospital called David had visited Adam at home to have a chat with him about his diet, the exercise classes, and eventually returning back to work. He also gave Adam an appointment to come into hospital to use the treadmill. This checked how well his heart was working. After a heart attack the heart is scarred;

it does not repair itself completely so exercise is extremely important to get it back into shape.

Adam enjoyed the classes; a ten minute warm up, then vigorous exercise, then ten minute warm down. Each time the pulse is taken, at rest then during exercise. Most of the patients were men and older than Adam except one guy, he had worked on Meridian television. His problem had been a virus that affected his heart. Most of the class had recognised him from the telly, Adam included.

The classes gave Adam back his confidence and the reassurance that these were making his heart stronger gave him even more confidence about his recovery. He could also talk to the other class members who had been through similar ordeals.

He attended his check-up in the hospital and passed the treadmill test with flying colours. This gave Adam an even bigger confidence boost, he was told by the lady doctor, 'You only have one heart, look after it'

It is something he has never forgotten.

Because Adam was home and back driving we were then able to take Diana in our car to her counsellor appointments. It wasn't stressful for Adam as we would go to the restaurant and have a cup of tea while we waited for Diana. After one of her appointments she came out crying and very distressed, her eyes wide and frightened. I couldn't understand what she was trying to tell me, so I gave her a piece of paper and asked she write it down, she wrote brain scan. I told her not to worry but deep down it really did worry me. What were they thinking of? Was there something that had been missed? A tumour? Is that why her speech was bad? I spoke to her counsellor Ellen by phone later on that day. She told me they wanted to refer her to a speech therapist, but before that they wanted her to have a brain scan to check there was nothing else that was affecting her speech. Just as I had thought. I asked many questions, and the one thing I was worrying about; were they thinking along the lines of a tumour? She told me that yes they had to rule that out before they went on to the next step. Please, God give us a break!

With so much to think about my sleep was badly affected as lying in bed at night I went from one person to the next. My mum also, as even though she was in between treatments none of us knew the outcome. I tossed and turned so my only choice was to watch T.V. until I couldn't keep my eyes open. Sometimes I saw two o'clock, three o'clock. I tried reading as well but I was never asleep before one a.m. I felt so irritable in the mornings and could hardly get myself out of bed, for the same routine to start all over again, not knowing that it was to get very much worse.

Adam's boss had told him not to come back to work until after Christmas which was good of him, as Adam could have returned after six weeks. It was nice having him home and I could look after him and keep an eye on him.

When he did finally go back I worried again as to how he would cope, but he was fine seeing his old customers and keeping busy did him good; he had no more panic attacks and carried on as usual. He had lost quite a bit of weight, which he looked good for doing so, and he needed a belt to keep his trousers up! Many of his customers had rung in to his head office concerned, as his answer phone calls were being diverted to his work colleague whilst he was off work. In the end Adam's boss had to send out emails to them, as many were ringing in saying they were concerned that they couldn't get hold of him. Rumours were rife. Adam is very well liked and it was like Chinese whispers. It went from he had left and gone back to his old company, to heart attack and worse. So the email was to stop all the speculation. Many customers sent cards and well wishes to head office which were then forwarded on to him, so going back to work he had a lot of people to thank and probably tell the same story for the hundredth time.

Chapter 9

It was about February time when I noticed a change in Diana's looks. It is difficult to describe but her facial features looked different, (a sort of blank faraway look is the only way to describe it) and when you spoke to her she didn't always grasp what you were saying, almost staring right through you while nodding her head up and down. Other days she was ok; she still had the speech problems, the corners of her mouth looked like they were drooping slightly. I began to feel I was imagining things as no two days were the same. She had come to me one day really sobbing, she had cried many times before but this again was different. I could tell she was very frightened about something, but she couldn't tell me what was upsetting her so much. She had written down on a piece of paper, 'I haven't spoken and my breath smells.'

Tears were streaming down her face, she sobbed and was inconsolable. Right there and then I made an appointment to see a doctor. She needed help as this situation with her was going on far too long, I really didn't know how to handle it. If it scared me, how must the children be feeling living with it every day? Nothing was improving; it was frightening for her and getting worse day by day.

I told the doctor about her speech and her breath and that she seemed very distressed and how worried we all were about her continuing decline. I explained about her blank expression and how she had altered so much in every way; looks, behaviour, everything I could think of I said it. And the counselling sessions that didn't seem to be helping. It all came out in one big gush so I didn't forget anything. Hearing it all Diana started to cry again. The doctor did a few tests. He poked a long stick thing into her mouth to check her gagging reflexes. I could see for myself that these were fine and then he told Diana that because her speech was bad and that not using her voice was probably why her breath smelt, and the best thing was to gargle every day to help it. He told me he would refer Diana to see a doctor at the Ears, Nose and Throat Unit to get her throat and vocal cords checked. I must admit I felt so much better after seeing him and Diana looked a little easier and less distressed when we left. If the doctor wasn't worried then it must be ok. I bought her some mouthwash and said that she wasn't to worry about herself and that her appointment wouldn't be long. Thinking back now while life is a bit quieter I'm wondering if I could have been more, I can only think of the word patient. Don't get me wrong I never shouted at her or got cross but I wanted things back to normal but normal they weren't and they were getting worse not better. If only I had known then how ill she was becoming then maybe before the Dementia set in I could have hugged her more and reassured her; hindsight would be so useful in times like these. I love all my family to bits but patience is something I struggle with, I've always wanted things done yesterday and not tomorrow. And I have never been a cuddler; my children yes when they were little but never a hugger of grown-ups! I always thought it soppy.

And because I worry so I want problems sorted pronto. Diana had a problem and I wanted it sorted, her well again, things how they were. Her need of my help was great and very, very time consuming. As a child I was very independent, never liked a fuss and got things done quickly so I had more time for other things.

Chapter 10

As if life wasn't tough enough, yet another event took place just to add to the never-ending problems. (Why not chuck it all at us?!) My dad had been complaining of back pain; in fact he had been complaining of back pain on and off for nearly two years. He refused point-blank to go to the doctors (he hates going) and announced that 'those white tablets he once took would do the trick'. The tablets in question were Ibuprofen. I had offered to take him to our out-of-hours doctors at the hospital but he wouldn't go.

'No. I'll be fine it's only backache,' he said.

But mum would ring me and say, 'You're dad's back must be bad today because he doesn't want any dinner.'

This is how he went on but to be honest I had enough to think about and I couldn't deal with a stubborn pensioner. I couldn't make him have a check-up and only a hammer over the head would get him there. And I wasn't going to be the one to hit him! That I decided was Mum's job! Until, that is, 1st March 2009 when the decision was taken out of his hands. It was my Mum and Dad's 50th wedding anniversary. I had been at home nursing a really bad throat and the start of a cough (one of my bugbears whenever I got a cold I got a bad cough). I had stayed home feeling pretty lousy, when the phone rang. It was Mum. 'I've phoned for an ambulance. Can you come?' I knew straight away it was Dad and his back. Adam and I rushed to their home. Dad looked dreadful; he was holding his side, he looked clammy, his hair was damp and his face was a yellow grey colour.

'How're you feeling, Dad?' I asked. (Silly question.)

'Not too good, pet,' he replied. 'It's my back. It's hurting like hell.'

He looked like a dead man walking as the sweat poured from him. The ambulance arrived quite quickly and checked him over thoroughly.

'His heart seems fine, his colour is a bit off, and he's a bit clammy.' I personally thought he looked like he would die any minute.

'I think we'll send for the doctor just to check him over and perhaps you can take him to the surgery in the week.'

'But he looks awful,' I said. 'I'll never get him there.'

'Well his blood pressure is fine, his heart rate is steady.'

'But what about his back pain?'

'Don't worry. If the doctor thinks he needs to go in we'll come back.'

With that it took half an hour to do the paper work, longer than it took to examine my dad. Don't get me wrong, I think paramedics are wonderful but my dad looked seriously ill. With that they left. My dad seemed calmer and his breathing was steady but he still looked awful. So we waited for the doctor and I can honestly say this brilliant guy saved my dad's life. He was a South African doctor called Doctor van Ryan and thank God whilst he was checking my dad over he asked him if he could manage a urine sample. I helped him to the downstairs loo, after a few minutes I thought I had better check on him as he hadn't yet reappeared. As I got to the door my dad opened it and there before me stood someone I can only describe as as near to death as could be. As soon as Doctor Van Ryan saw him he said, 'Quick we've got to lay him down. I know what this is, it's an Aortic Aneurism.' As soon as we laid Dad down his colour started to return and his breathing became less laboured. His colour was still grey/yellow even tinged with green. I can tell you I have never been so scared in my life and the admiration I felt for this doctor is indescribable.

He called the ambulance back and the only thing I kept thinking was if the doctor hadn't have come my dad would have got up to go to bed later on and collapsed and died. And that is exactly what Doctor van Ryan told us would have happened. I asked him how he knew what my dad had and he explained that he had witnessed exactly the same thing once before and recognised the symptoms as soon as my dad came out of the toilet. All I can say is he was obviously meant to be on call that night to save my dad's life. It obviously wasn't my dad's turn to meet his maker. Dr Van Ryan rang the hospital, he said that he felt the only place to deal with this was the John Radcliff in Oxford, so my dad was placed into the ambulance, wheeled out at an angle re Dr van Ryan's instructions as it prevented more leakage. 'God, what a guy!'

When they left with my dad he told us to follow on in a little while as he needed information. He laughed when we told him he hadn't seen a doctor in forty years due to his fear. I asked what caused his aneurism. He asked, 'Did he smoke?'

'Yes but he hasn't smoked since we were teenagers.'

'The damage had already been done,' he replied. 'The leak would have been very slow and not enough to bother him, but now it had become more serious and that is why these past two years he had been complaining of back pain and ignoring it with pain killers.' Typical of my father; hates the doctors, will have his flu jab every year but ignores bad back pain!

Mum got together his things. By now it was ten p.m. and she looked shattered so we told her to stay home. Once again Adam and I set off to another hospital. I was feeling pretty ill myself as I was continuously sucking sweets to stop my cough and I was in a sort of daze as what the hell was going on with my family to deserve all this. We got to casualty pretty quick as at that time of night the roads were very quiet except for the odd lorry.

We were taken to see my dad as soon as we arrived. He was in a little cubicle, he didn't seem too bad. He actually looked a lot better than previously as I had no idea what to expect when we saw him. I held his hand. 'You ok, Dad?'

'Yes, pet,' he said. 'Hope I don't get that MRSA,' he said.

'Well don't get it,' I said, trying to make a joke. It made him laugh.

'My will,' he said and he started mumbling about me and my sisters and if he didn't survive…

Again I joked, 'Well how many daughters have you got then?' I teased him. 'You didn't have a bike did you? Have I got other siblings then?'

'No just you two.'

'Well stop worrying, Dad and just rest.'

Again he started to chatter on. Definitely nerves. Dad always jokes when he's nervous, same as me I suppose. I think he was trying to tell me about his will and where to find things, but he wasn't making sense. Suddenly beside me appeared a doctor. 'Can I speak to you for a minute?'

I followed him outside the cubicle and out of my dad's earshot. 'I'm afraid it's pretty serious. It's a six inch aneurism; the biggest I've ever seen. Your father may not survive this.'

My heart started pounding but for some reason I wasn't worried. I don't know why, but hadn't Dr Van Ryan already saved him at home? It wasn't meant to be the end of my dad, I just knew it. I went back to my dad and kissed his cheek and told him I'd see him later. 'Ok, pet, see you later.' And I knew deep down I would.

We watched him go as they wheeled him to the theatre. I felt such total shock, this just couldn't be happening. What had my family done to warrant such hurt and heartache? I felt I couldn't take much more of this. Adam put his hand on my shoulder. 'He'll be fine I'm sure of it.'

I couldn't even cry, I was all cried out, I felt drained and I felt like screaming 'Why? Haven't we been through enough?' I looked about me. There were other people in the cubicles; a woman mopping her husband's brow, he was attached to a monitor; a boy with a plaster on his leg and a tear stained face; a small child crying while her mother tried to calm her down. Were these people having a crap year like us? I could ask but they'd think I was potty! 'Excuse me are you all having a crap year like us?'

I pulled myself together and went to find a phone to call my mum. By now it was nearly midnight. I told her the truth and what the doctor had said and then I started to cry. What if he was right and my dad did die? My mum sounded choked and then said to go and get a cup of tea and that she was sure they would do everything they could to save Dad's life. My head was pounding and I was running out of sweets to suck. I told her I would ring as soon as I knew anything then hung up. We made our way to the café on the next floor. The only person there was a lady sat at a table with a load of paper work spread about her. 'Can we still get a cup of tea?' I asked.

'Yeah, we're open till two,' the lady replied drolly, looking quite annoyed and very unfriendly because we had disturbed her work, obviously something to do with the café. Adam got two teas and a bottle of cold drink for my cough. I didn't want any food as I was feeling sick with worry, and sick from coughing. I was starting to feel very hot and quite unwell as my throat was sore from coughing, and my head ached from the heat in the hospital, the germs must love multiplying in places like this. We sat there for ages not sure what time to go back to the waiting room. We talked things over. I wasn't even surprised at what had happened I was just so worn out and in total disbelief that my dad should become ill so soon after Adam's heart attack. I was told once that these things happen and problems seem to come one after the other. Well, boy, it was going that way for us. I held the cold coke can to my hot aching head and after rummaging through my complete mess of a handbag I found two Paracetamol, oh joy!

We made our way downstairs after about an hour. We went and sat down in the larger, cooler waiting room we had seen as we had first entered the hospital. There was a huge T.V. on the wall; it was on but there was no sound. Why do they do that? What's the point of turning it on and leaving it on mute? It wouldn't have bothered anyone with the volume up slightly. I sat there looking at the screen trying to lip read. No, I couldn't lip read so that was that. I looked around the room. A lady sat texting on her phone; a young boy had his head on an older lady's shoulders, his mother I presumed; a man in a wheelchair with blood on a shoeless foot. I remember thinking what could he have possibly been doing in the early hours of the morning? He looked too old to have been out drinking with his mates and got into trouble. Had he been decorating barefoot and dropped the paint tin on his foot? Perhaps his dog had been sleeping on the end of his bed and bit his foot? I laughed at myself for thinking that, as our dog slept on the bed and often growled when we shoved him over. But probably the most logical answer was he had been waiting in casualty for ages and was still waiting to be seen.

Suddenly a nurse appeared next to me. 'I've been looking for you two.'

I froze as I prepared myself for the worst. 'Would you like to come and wait in the family room? It's much more comfortable, you can make some tea if you like.'

'Oh yes, yes,' I said relieved. 'Have you heard anything yet?' I asked.

'No but the doctor will come and see you as soon as they have finished operating on your dad. She showed us to the family room, and then she left.

We sat watching the telly or sort of watching it. It was nice to sit on something comfortable, but the room was very stuffy which wouldn't help my cough. Still it was better to be there than on the uncomfortable chairs in the waiting room.

There were two large black soft leather settees, a coffee table and a kitchen area to make a drink. I could see Adam was having trouble keeping his eyes open as it was now two a.m., and since he had suffered his heart attack he got tired very quickly. I kept sipping my drink to stop my cough and popping cherry flavoured cough sweets in my mouth every time I finished one.

So many thoughts went through my head. I thought about the time I went to see a clairvoyant. She described my father as a Jekyll and Hyde character. 'Can be a bit of a comedian.' Yep, that was true. 'He has a rather large handlebar moustache.' Yep correct again, but she didn't tell me about this. Apparently clairvoyants are not allowed to say anything distressing so if she had seen this happening she wouldn't have told me. 'You have a fear of cancer.' Correct! 'Your mother and father will one day live in a bungalow.' Not quite right. The house they are in now had a garage, which was converted into a sitting room for my mother! 'One day you'll write a book.' Ah, didn't know about that. I quite liked English and I loved reading but what would I have written about, until now that is! Did she really see all that had happened? I will never know or even understand how mediums have these skills or gifts. She said so much more which a lot has been so accurate. She was very well known and I saw her twice. Sadly the lady in question died. I'm sure she saw it coming and cancelled her future sittings!

At about 2.30 a.m. we heard footsteps coming along the corridor. My heart began to thump in my chest, I had felt like this when Adam had his heart attack and here I was again waiting to hear if another member of my family was going to be ok. A young doctor entered the room and sat down facing me; we were almost touching knees. 'Well I'm pleased to tell you your dad is ok, everything went well. It was a six inch aneurism, the largest I have ever operated on. I'm very surprised he made it, he must be a very strong man. He will be in ICU for a few days. You can come and see him but he will be kept sedated so he can recover.' I let out an enormous sigh.

'Can we visit him tomorrow?' I asked.

'Yes but he will be sleeping so don't expect too much for the first few days.'

I thanked him and we wearily made our way back to the car. The fresh air was fantastically reviving. I couldn't wait to get home and into bed. I phoned my mum from our mobile it was now 3.45 a.m. but I knew she wouldn't be sleeping. By now I was nearly hoarse from my coughing; I knew my mum felt bad that Adam and I were at yet another hospital. We had actually joked once that we should buy a house right next to the hospital then whoever was due in could stay the night with us and I could walk them round in the morning. It's a good job we both have a very good sense of humour. I think anyone else would have jumped off a tall building by now! I could hear from her voice she was relieved, I told her I would ring her in the morning.

It was very difficult to sleep as we were now very over tired and all I did was yawn and then cough so in the end I came downstairs and made a cup of tea, propped myself up on our settee and sat watching some soppy old film on Sky. I must have dozed off as I was woken by our Jack Russell jumping on me; it was now 7 a.m. Adam was already up he made us tea. The way I was feeling I knew I wouldn't be able to visit my dad and I knew that being unwell I would not be allowed in ICU in case I spread my germs. So luckily my son John and his wife Chloe volunteered to take my mum into see Dad as Adam had a very busy day at work and it would have been so unfair that he then had to arrive home from work and then go straight out again. They left home before the rush hour and got to Dad at about five o'clock. I had rung earlier that day to see how he was doing and amazingly Dad was already awake and sat by his bed and had sent one of the nurses to fetch him a paper to read. So from being told he would be sedated in intensive care to sitting by his bed giving orders was so like my dad. I laughed when the nurse told me, 'Your father is doing so well it is incredible.'

'He must be very strong, and determined,' I added.

He was still in intensive care when they got there but he was cracking jokes just like he always does. His nurses had to stay with him at all times; he was wired up to machines just as Adam had been and had blood pressure checked frequently through the day. In all, my dad stayed in hospital for five days and I bet it was the noisiest time they had ever experienced. I couldn't see him until the day he was due home as I felt unwell for the rest of that week.

The hospital sent him home with two walking frames so he could walk safely to the loo etc. Luckily my parents have an upstairs and downstairs loo so once Dad was downstairs he could stay put until bedtime. He did look so much better than I had seen him in a long time. He had a good colour and his appetite was so much better now. And he was pain free, only sore from his operation and that was manageable. His recovery was amazing and he had more energy. It makes me cringe to think of the days he rode his bike as he did most days down to the shops to fetch his paper and any shopping needed by our mum. What if he had taken ill and fallen into the road and been run over?

That's why I know it wasn't his time to kick the bucket. If he had allowed me to take him to the doctors when he first felt unwell it may never have come to this, but Dad is incredibly stubborn and incredibly lucky to be alive!

Chapter 11

At last Diana's Ear, Nose and Throat appointment came through. We picked her up at about ten a.m. as her appointment was at eleven a.m. The traffic was always unpredictable so it was always best to leave an hour for the journey. She was very subdued that day and probably weary as we all were from constant consultations but never getting to the solution. Maybe today something would show up. Poor girl was on the verge of tears and so much thinner these days. I spoke to her about anything that came into my head to try and relax her and admittedly her having the barest of speech it was so difficult, I just kept chatting on as the quiet was so freaky. Diana and I could always chat for England but I honestly felt uncomfortable. I know I was waffling like a demented idiot.

Sometimes I wondered if she actually heard me or even took it in whilst I repeated myself twice on many occasions.

Please find a way back, Diana!

We didn't have to wait as long as I had anticipated, as Ear Nose and Throat is usually packed, but today it was nearly empty. 'Thank you; thank you,' I said to myself. I just really wanted to be home. I think perhaps in my next life I will come back as a nurse or doctor at a local hospital, as I seem to spend so much time sat in one!

It wasn't long before they called Diana's name. I explained I needed to come in because of her speech.

The doctor, a really friendly, smiley guy, sat her down in front of him and explained to us both what he was going to do. Diana began to cry as she did many times these days. We both comforted her; she blew her nose then sat as good as gold. He sprayed her throat to numb it then he slowly fed a camera through her nose. She didn't like it and kept moving. The doctor was very good with her and kept talking. 'If you stay still, Diana it will be over very quickly.' She did as he requested. I could see Diana's throat as clear as day on a screen. Nothing abnormal he said, no nodules or lumps or growths. Diana cried again after he removed the camera. This was so upsetting for her. He said everything seemed fine.

This was all so frustrating especially for my sister. Appointment after appointment and still no nearer to a diagnosis. How the hell was this going to end?

Once we had got back to the car Diana seemed to forget her ordeal and stared blankly out of the car window. Seemingly unaffected by her ordeal thank goodness. Another appointment to strike off the ever-growing list.

Don't get me wrong, I always tried to reassure Diana as best I could even though I found all this hard work I would never have wished this on anyone and knowing the old Diana she would have been the first to admit all this was a pain in the arse.

I was missing the old Diana, the one I could talk to if I had a problem, always the first to help if she could. We knew a lady called Janet. She lived very near me; she was a seamstress and used to alter Liam's school trousers for Diana. Whenever she saw us together she used to sing 'sisters, sisters there were never such devoted sisters'. I was missing all that as we were together a lot and now people were noticing that we weren't and asking where she was when they met me without her. It became difficult to explain and very long winded so in the end I just said she wasn't feeling too good and left it at that. I didn't want to keep telling the story, it was our business no one else's.

This Diana was like a stranger that I didn't know. Yeah, she looked like her, except the weight loss was noticeable. She lived at the same address, but it wasn't her. The old Diana I could talk about anything, the old Diana was always up for a laugh.

Like the time we were walking home from the shops one morning. Along the road came a, well I can only call him a midget/dwarf, we knew him slightly, but never his name. We had chatted to him many times as he worked at the supermarket we had just left collecting trolley's. A nice chap and very friendly, he came straight up to me and asked if I would mind doing up his trouser belt as he hadn't had any help that morning to get dressed (his arms were typically short, and his small hands couldn't cope with buckles etc.) Well him being so short I had to kneel down in front of him to locate the belt under his little pot belly. My head bent downwards to see what I was doing. All I could hear were cars tooting and my sister squawking with laughter ahead of me. Apparently to her and probably to passers-by it looked like I was giving a dwarf a blow job – on the main street, with loads of cars passing close by. She laughed all the way home (and for many days afterwards). I caught up with her red faced wondering who had been in the cars that had tooted at us.

'That looked so funny and bloody filthy,' she added. She then told everyone in the school playground later that day.

I can tell you if ever I saw him coming I hid until he went past, as Diana started giggling as soon as she saw him.

I just wished that we could go back to those happier daft, unpredictable days, to turn the clock back to when Diana was her old self. She had never been a moody person, and we never missed a day phoning each other, to chat, gossip and moan; now this never happened. She was always content at home cooking and doing her housework. As for me I never knew what mood I would be in from one day to the next. Maybe it's because I am a Gemini, a person with many personalities? Although all the different things that happened each day, and believe me every day was eventful, made me miserable. It is difficult to stay calm and not be reduced to tears when you are being bombarded with letters and problems and tears and appointments and none of them are yours. I usually cope with whatever is thrown at me but some days I just wanted to throw them right back!

One incident that happened which triggered more alarm bells in the counsellor's head was one warm day, morning I think, Diana suddenly appeared at my house. She came in with a big smile on her face she couldn't explain herself. She was trying to tell me something, so I gave her a piece of paper to write on. The exact words she wrote were 'there's a boy in summerhouse'. I looked at her confused.

'Do you mean someone's got into the garden?' She nodded.

I quickly rang her home and Liam answered. 'I've got your mum here, Liam. Is there someone in the garden, a boy?'

'I dunno,' came the reply. 'You're freaking me out, Aunty Jan.'

'Look just stay in the house and I'll be straight over,' I said.

Luckily James had just turned up from work so he took us over there. Diana rushed straight into the garden and started looking into the summerhouse. I checked inside myself and inside the shed. I could see my reflection in the glass. 'I think you saw your reflection in the glass, Diana, don't you?' But she continued to look as if whatever it was she had seen was real and it had frightened her.

'I think she really saw something, Mum,' James said to me quietly so that Diana didn't hear. Her garden fence backed onto another house. Was it possible that a boy had climbed over and scared her?

'Did someone come over the fence, Diana?' She looked at me and nodded. 'Did they run off then?' She nodded again. I shuddered as this was so weird. 'Look, whoever it was must have run off. Come on,' I said, 'let's go to Mum's for a cup of tea.'

I couldn't think what else to do. It was pointless phoning the police as there was nothing they could do. So off we went to our mother's. Diana came quite happily, sitting at our mother's she seemed to forget what had happened. This was freaky, so I didn't mention it again. But the next day, a Saturday she appeared again at my house at about one p.m. She wrote down exactly the same thing. She kept smiling at me like she was being mischievous. Adam could see my annoyance as I really felt she was doing this for attention. How wrong was I?! I didn't know it but this was the beginning of the Dementia.

Adam said, 'Come on, Diana, let's go and look again.' So off we all went and again she looked inside and out of the summerhouse as if searching for someone her eyes wide and frightened and she kept pointing at the door. I could see it was freaking out the kids so I said, 'I know would you all like to come to footy today and watch the boys play?' I could see Liam and Lauren were relieved to have something to do as this was very strange behaviour and not something we had experienced before. Diana seemed happy to get away from the house. Boy this was getting more and more weird. None of this was making any sense so I decided to call Ellen her counsellor on the Monday to tell her what had occurred as this was really strange behaviour and had not happened before. Ellen didn't say too much then but later on explained that it had rung alarm bells in her head. Ellen said she would chase up Diana's appointment.

At last in early April Diana received her appointment to have a brain scan. Were they now looking for a tumour? This was becoming more frightening by the day. I think it was a CT scan. This didn't show anything. Thank God it wasn't a brain tumour or such like as I had feared. Another appointment bit the dust!

Lauren usually had to intercept much of Diana's mail now, as she tended to hide it away, or take it to our mum which mum then gave to me to deal with, if not then Diana brought it straight round to me. Whatever mail came she just didn't want it in the house, this too became one of her peculiar habits. I would open it, reassure her that I would deal with the letter later, as by now she was usually in floods of tears over anything that was pushed through her letterbox. Any mail really upset her so I would put the offending letters to one side out of her view, this then calmed her down. Again I put it down to some kind of depression, what else could it be? I had no explanation for this strange behaviour.

It got so my heart would thump every time I heard the gate go click as I was finding it freaky and difficult to get my head around Diana's peculiar routine.

One hospital letter arrived which luckily Lauren had opened and read to me. It read, 'Dear Mrs Parsons, as you have missed your February appointment with Doctor Bolton could you please let us know if you still require to see him.' I immediately rang to say that Diana had never received a letter with an appointment for February and that yes could she have one as soon as possible. They assured me that one had definitely been sent but they apologised in case it had been lost in the post. The missing letter I found much later was hidden in the back of one of Diana's drawers. Diana had obviously hidden it away.

I assumed the counsellors at Beech Croft, Ellen and her team must have requested this appointment with Doctor Bolton, he was part of the Neurological team.

We saw Doctor Bolton about 16th April. He did lots of tests on Diana. He asked her to look at pictures, and copy them and write down what she saw. She had to point to things as he asked her, to tie up the pictures with the writing. I could see she was having trouble and took a long time to complete everything he requested. It felt like sitting in a classroom. He took her in a side room and asked her to undress. Lauren had to help her as for quite a while she had become weaker in her arms. Again another sign we mistook for something else. Maybe if all the other things going on hadn't happened, I might have noticed more and kept on at her doctors, but I was running two homes and looking after money and shopping and dealing with much correspondence and attending Mum's treatment which had begun again. Don't get me wrong, I would never have not gone with Mum but I was feeling so tired and angry that no one seemed to know what was wrong with my sister.

If I had been Superman I may have coped better but all I wanted were answers that nobody seemed to able to give me.

After her tests I remember clearly and so probably does Lauren, how Doctor Bolton snapped our heads off. His words were, 'This is more than just depression, there is something more serious going on here.'

The only thing I could think of to say was, 'We didn't know, it all happened when her husband left.' Which sounded so pathetic and dumb, when I said it but he had no idea what had been happening to our family. I didn't have time to explain everything and to be honest I'm sure he didn't want to hear it, his concern was for Diana and rightly so. But I came away feeling I had failed my sister somehow and we still didn't know what was wrong. He obviously had an idea but wanted Diana to be seen at the John Radcliff Hospital in Oxford.

12th May 2009 will be another date that will stay firmly fixed in my head, it was the day we found out my sister's fate. I can honestly say that it was the last thing I ever expected to be told. We arrived at the hospital at about nine a.m. Me, Diana and her ever faithful Lauren. I'm not saying that Liam isn't just as faithful but his learning difficulties make it hard for him to cope with so many of life's challenges. His father's leaving was one, his mother's illness another, he would stutter when he couldn't cope with certain situations and sitting in a hospital room seeing his mother have various tests would have been extremely hard for Liam to deal with. Things had to be explained to Liam in a certain way in order for him to cope with them and understand.

The first test was a machine that tested Diana's muscles. I didn't understand why they were doing it but I knew they were testing for something specific. I felt sure that they were going to say it was a complete nervous breakdown. The test took about twenty minutes, Diana had wires placed on strategic areas of her legs and ankles. These were attached to a machine which took readings, I guessed it was to test how well her muscles were working. I could see wiggly lines and heard a few bleeps coming from the machine, that is the only way I can describe the test.

Diana calmly sat on the bed appearing not to care that she was wired up. We were then told to return to the ward and a consultant would see her shortly. It was by now nearly lunchtime and we were starving. The whole time Diana kept staring at me with frightened wide eyes, no longer calm in appearance as she was a few minutes before. To be honest I didn't know what to say to her or how to reassure her. I felt guilty that she was ill and I admit I found it hard meeting her eyes. She looked to me for help and answers, none of which I had. I just wished the consultants would hurry up and then we could go home.

Lauren and I decided to play eye spy as we were so bored sat there. I also made up a game which made her giggle, we had to hum a pop song and guess the tune which isn't easy to do and neither of us got very many right, but it took some of the boredom away and it made Lauren giggle because of its silliness. I then went downstairs and got us some food, as the nurse had brought some lunch to Diana's bed. So that meant the doctors were probably having their lunch. At about 2.30 several doctors came to Diana's bed they asked her to lie down while they carried out more tests. They asked her to push as hard as she could with her hands against the consultant's hand, then her arms against his hands, then they asked her to move her tongue as fast as she could side to side; that she found difficult. I understood a few things they said, things like weakness in her arms and weakness in her tongue. The rest of it was doctors' language. One of the doctors, I think he was the head consultant, asked Diana to write down what year it was. She wrote down after some thought 2008 and not 9. When was Lauren's birthday? Again she looked like she was thinking very hard. She wrote down 16th September 2008. Her birthday is in fact in October. Diana couldn't even remember what day of the week it was, most things requested of her were incorrect.

He asked Lauren and I several things. When did we notice Diana began to alter? We both agreed. 'About four months after her husband walked out. Diana altered in behaviour and speech first, and then slowly in appearance,' I told him.

At the end of the tests and questions the head consultant asked we accompany him into a side room. He asked if Lauren wanted to be in the room with us. Straight away this rang alarm bells in my head; this was going to be bad. How bad I was just about to find out. He started to speak. 'I'm very sorry to say but Diana has Motor Neurone and frontal lobe

Dementia. The two have crossed over; it is very rare to have the two together.'

The words that rang in my ears were Motor Neurone. I knew Lauren didn't know what it was; Lauren started firing questions at him. I didn't need to, I knew exactly how bad it was. As for Diana, I'm not sure if she knew what it meant or even understood as she didn't cry, until Lauren started to cry because he said, 'Unfortunately there is No treatment, and No cure.' I just sat there in total utter shock, I had just been hit by a speeding train, my body was covered in goose bumps as I tried to hold it together. My lovely, kind, once beautiful sister had just been given a death sentence. When he asked if we had any questions I honest to God couldn't think of one. There wasn't a thing I could ask to improve my sister's outcome. She was going to die and I had no idea how soon that might be. He continued to talk to us but I can honestly say I didn't hear another word. Motor Neurone kept flashing in my head. And what could I possibly ask him in front of Lauren? I couldn't discuss Diana's imminent death, how long had she got etc.? That would have been too cruel.

I needed to get them home and now.

We left his room in total silence, the day was warm and the sunshine was reviving, but it meant nothing. Unbelievably Diana seemed to completely forget what he had just said; she didn't request to write anything down to ask questions.

As anyone else being dealt that hand would have gone to pieces, I truly believe her Dementia saved her heartbreak and the true knowledge of what her fate now was. They say God works in mysterious ways and I thanked God in his wisdom for her Dementia, she didn't remember what had been told to her, or she didn't understand it. She didn't know she was going to leave her precious children, which for any mother would be an absolute tragedy. Thinking back now I believe that Diana only cried because Lauren did, I don't think she really understood what the consultant had told us. I have read up on the symptoms and Diana's type of Dementia is associated with Motor Neurone, it explains that a person can become distracted and withdrawn and also have compulsive behaviour. Such as in Diana's case she was constantly walking backwards and forwards to the kitchen looking in the fridge for food, or repeatedly opening and closing doors and windows. She didn't like anything moved; everything had to stay the same.

And she would become cross if food was taken away from her. It all became so clear, her inability to empathise with others, her blank looks, lack of affection towards the children and she would just cry for no reason. So much fell into place now. And her speech that I believed was caused by shock, which had become bad so very early on, was never going to come back. It would get worse until she could make no sound at all. I knew all about this bloody disease. I had seen a play once and a documentary all about the awful way it ravages your body. I remember how the documentary had made me feel sad that something so terrible existed and now my sister had it. Fuck! Fuck!

We travelled home in complete silence. Adam could tell by the look I gave him that it was serious and not to ask anything. Diana just looked out of the window with no expression or emotion. Thank God for the Dementia. Lauren sat cuddled up next to her mum. And as for me I couldn't think of a thing to talk about which is very unusual for me, but the wind had well and truly been taken from my sails, so I put on the car radio to break the silence. I didn't hear a thing apart from me repeating in my head oh my God Motor Neurone why?! Please NOT my sister! This just couldn't be happening it happened to other people! And I couldn't cry, even though I felt like screaming I couldn't, not until I was home away from them both and when I started I knew I wouldn't stop.

We called into our mum's on the way home. I couldn't say anything to her at first as Diana picked up that I was trying to tell Mum something, she followed me into the kitchen and started to cry as she was aware of something serious being discussed. I whispered to Mum I would ring her when I got home. Diana sat and drank her tea forgetting again what she had heard in the kitchen. A blank look on her face.

Now things really began to change, my attitude and feeling sorry for myself for one thing. This illness was something

Diana would need as much help as possible with. My stress had to take a back seat; she would need me more than ever now so it was onwards and upwards.

Take each day as it comes and deal with problems as they arise was the only way to survive this. My heart was broken and I couldn't imagine life without Diana in it.

I felt terrified. I knew how bad this would become and the last thing I wanted was for my sister to suffer. At the moment she wasn't too bad but what about later on? How would we all cope? How would I cope? I know I'd have to dig deep into my reserve; if I had any that is!

At first things could stay relatively the same although I watched her like a hawk as we carried on much as normal. Lauren went to school and saw her friends as much as possible. Liam still had no job; it wasn't a priority at the moment. But to this day there has been nothing suitable for him and his disabilities. Or the jobs he may be able to do were already taken. I never did agree with us joining the common market. I remember my dad saying back in the '70s that Enoch Powell had got it right, that we are just a small country and letting in so many immigrants would lead to a crisis. Eventually there will be a lack of jobs for the people that were born and live in the UK. Enoch's prediction was so right he had the hindsight others chose to ignore. I'm not racist but we live on a small island that probably only has enough jobs for the people that live on it. Letting in too many people is heading for mass unemployment. So many people are on benefits when there should be enough jobs to go round. This government needs another Margaret Thatcher, or even an Enoch Powell (tough, no nonsense people). Our politicians are too busy claiming on second houses, poodles being clipped, pools being cleaned and arguing with each other, why not work together for the sake of our country, a coalition.

No wonder people all head here, hiding on ships and on lorries. Free healthcare and benefits. I was shocked to read a family housed in a large luxury London house, the rent being paid for by the councils, it is utterly laughable. I have to find a home for my niece and nephew perhaps they will get a seven bedroom mansion for nothing? I doubt it!!

We need to be more like Australia; if you have something to offer, a trade or skill then we'll see. I don't hear anyone complaining about Australia not doing their bit, they are protecting their own! But in our case soft old UK it's come one come all, take our houses, take our jobs and take our benefits! The latest figures 1st July 2011, there are 62.5 million people living in our country, if we don't go carefully we will sink! (Might ask my joiner son to start building an ark.)

I feel sorry for the poorer countries and their poverty but as a country can we take on everyone else's problems? There is only so much we can do. We should look out for ourselves first then offer assistance (if we can afford to) where it is needed. As a whole we help as much as we can, things like Children in Need and Red Nose Day, Sport Relief and various charities. These things are brilliant, and we are the first to help out when there is some kind of catastrophe elsewhere in the world.

So finding a job for Liam was never going to be easy but how many Liam's are there out there that could do with the help?

Unless you have good qualifications you don't have much hope of finding something with a good wage packet. Or hundreds are going after the same job. There are a lot of people who are of average intelligence and are not college/university material, myself included. In the seventies you left school and most of us kids got jobs without too much bother. Now kids leave school and find it hard to even find a suitable job or it takes a long time to find something that pays a decent wage.

Their only choice, sign on and wait for a job that may never come. Do employees give jobs to immigrants and pay them less? Yes I believe some do, so they are being exploited, and jobs aren't going to people from this country.

It is so definitely a case these days of not what you know but who you know. So how do people like Liam stand a chance? I hope one day someone gives him a job that not only pays him a decent wage but one suited to him. He receives disability living allowance but what kind of life does that give him? Just enough to scrape by. No life!

Adam and I decided not to book a holiday, as with Diana deteriorating and my mum still needing trips to the hospital it seemed selfish, so we carried on much the same.

Except my worry for Diana was even greater; I found myself watching her every move; the way she held her head; the way she had begun to lose weight. How much had she lost? I kept asking myself. Her walking seemed to slow up overnight. Her face looked gaunt and pale. And one thing that made me feel so incredibly sad was she started to carry a tissue around with her to wipe away her saliva; one of the common conditions of Motor Neurone is the uncontrollable dribbling.

Diana and Lauren would come over to my house every Saturday night and sometimes Fridays and we would all watch Ant and Dec and then X factor, our favourite programmes, and every so often I would glance over at Diana and she would be wiping her lips. My heart would practically break at the sight of this. I felt so angry at the Motor Neurone for doing this to her.

I wanted to sob my eyes out for her, but I couldn't. Not until I was alone that is.

Was this all brought on by the stress of Sean leaving? I will never know but seeing her like this made me want scream out loud and challenge the disease to a fight, to beat it out of her but it was all so hopeless. It was strong and was winning everyday that's what made me so angry. I had an awful choking feeling in my throat as I kept my feelings well hidden. All the time I was around them, I kept the humour going to make them laugh, although I didn't know how long Diana would be capable of enjoying a laugh. As how was the Dementia going to affect her later on we didn't know. It was very difficult to hold conversations anyway and I noticed she turned her head away from us and kept looking towards the telly because of course she could say nothing, nor comment on what we were watching and writing things down didn't make a lot of sense either. But I noticed she smiled when something funny was said and showed emotions in the right places. Or did she laugh because we did? How much she understood we didn't really know. If only it had been the dementia she had, and not both. I will never understand why. So much for someone so young. I felt deep down that she may never have got over her ex. Luckily the Dementia made her forget him. At least the children would still have had their mother with them, but why Motor Neurone as well? I won't ever understand and I will constantly ask 'Why?'

In June Diana had her first appointment with Professor Coles a specialist on Diana's illness; we also met her neurological nurse Claire whom I liked straight away.

Prof Coles asked me many questions about Diana and then she examined her. She asked her to lift her arms and roll her head, and open her mouth and roll her tongue, and all the time my poor sister unaware of so much smiled sweetly at Prof Coles. Thank God she didn't know how incredibly ill she was. I think she liked the attention and company and the ride out and as she wasn't aware of why she was being prodded and poked it didn't seem to bother her; she liked being with others.

We discussed with Prof Coles about the eventual need for carers. She told us she would request a lady called Jane to contact me from the social services disability unit, and that she also wanted someone from speech therapy to come and check Diana's swallowing regularly. She asked me about Diana's sleeping and her dribbling, and was she coping with the stairs? Was she managing to dress and undress? This I let Lauren answer and she told Prof Coles that her mum had trouble with jumpers and doing up her bra and that before going to school she helped her mum dress as Diana's arms had become weaker.

I was so pleased to hear Prof Coles say to Lauren that she was a credit to her mother, as I know she did a lot more than that. She hardly left her mother's side except to go to school and see friends occasionally. She and Liam became their mother's right arm, and this was only the beginning.

I know the two children had no idea how long their mother had to live and that Motor Neurone was such a cruel and terrible disease. And I wasn't going to ask in front of Lauren, I knew that it can be between two to five years, I prayed it was the latter as it would give them a few precious years with her. But deep down I had a feeling it wouldn't be as long as five. Her deterioration was so rapid.

Prof Coles said she wanted to see Diana again in September and that she would contact Diana's doctor to make her aware of Diana's condition, and that if there were any problems with her dribbling and sleeping then the doctor could prescribe something.

Within the next couple of weeks I received a phone call from someone called Jane. She explained a few things to me over the phone and said she would bring her colleague with her called Jack to meet us as he would be taking on Diana's case. Jack was the nicest guy I have ever met and the tallest; Jane was lovely, charming and softly spoken. They made me feel that we were in safe hands. They explained about claiming for Disability Living Allowance and because of that Diana's Employment and support would be increased. I was so pleased that at last they would have a bit more money, as Diana was desperate for underwear and because she had lost weight her clothes were very ill fitting and she desperately needed a warmer coat as she was feeling the cold more. And poor Lauren's school shoes had seen better days. I had spent so many times repairing Liam's jeans I think they spent more time with me than with him! Those would be first on the list along with the other items. These were all things that they needed. Until now they had very little to live on and I found myself giving them the odd tenner each, just so they could go and buy a few things they needed or even as in Lauren's case a much needed trip to the local cinema with her friends. To get her away from the problems they faced each day.

On Jane and Jack's first visit they told Lauren about the young carer's project. It arranged outings and getaway days, for children that care for adults. I could see by Lauren's face she wasn't keen; she said she would think about it. I think it was because at the time she didn't regard herself as a carer and this confused her a little. They also told us about things that could eventually help Diana around the home. One thing I pointed out straight away was that Diana was having trouble turning on one of the kitchen taps, as it was quite stiff. Diana had lost a lot of strength in her arms and hands. Jack told us that they had a company called Ridgeway that dealt with things like that in the home and that they would arrange for someone to come and change the taps, and as Diana was on benefits it wouldn't cost her anything. This company eventually became invaluable, as there were many aids Diana was to need as her illness took more and more hold. Thank goodness there are organisations like these to help with so many needs that arose as Diana's illness progressed.

Jack and Jane also discussed carers, which at the time we didn't even consider necessary, but they were both concerned because her Dementia would eventually make it dangerous for her to go out on her own; they wanted to know how she was coping with the roads etc.

At that time Diana only came over to me or straight round the corner to our mum's house. She had stopped going to the shops unless she was with someone as she couldn't make herself understood if she was spoken to and she couldn't ask for things she needed anymore. I also think she found it embarrassing if she bumped into people we knew who of course straight away realised something was wrong with her. She couldn't reply to them if they spoke to her. So eventually she only went out with her family and never alone.

It was agreed that I would call Jack as soon as we felt things were changing with Diana. He also suggested he call the Dementia team at Beech Croft at the Newbury hospital, to arrange for them to come along and meet us all and assess how Diana was coping with the Dementia and to see if they could offer support to Diana and ourselves. So began a tirade of frequent visitors; the speech therapist Sian was one of the first people to see Diana. She was a young Welsh girl whom Diana took to right away. Sian checked Diana's swallowing and made suggestions to make her swallowing easier. She told

Diana to hold her head high as she swallowed and not bend her head forward and to take small mouthfuls of food and small sips of drink. And this was the first time we were first introduced to Thick and Easy (or thick and squeezey as I called it).

It was to be added to Diana's drinks a small amount at first and to be increased when her swallowing became more difficult. Sian explained this in a matter of fact way, as she didn't want to scare Diana. I actually felt very scared though, as Diana's eating wasn't too bad at the moment so how bad would it become?

Sian demonstrated the marvels of Thick and Easy. It is to help the drink go down the throat and not straight into the lungs. (Motor Neurone sufferers usually die of breathing difficulties, usually pneumonia, the body becomes starved of oxygen and the patient dies)

I made Diana a cup of tea which I gave to Sian, so that she could add a sachet of the Thick and Easy to the cup. It was very funny as by the time she had stirred the mixture into the cup the spoon actually stood upright in Diana's cup.

'Yuk,' said Lauren.

'That looks like a cup of thick tar not tea,' I said. 'I think perhaps one of these sachets is a bit too much.' She laughed.

'When you get the tins on prescription, I think two scoops will suffice. It should be the consistency of custard so you may need to experiment a few times to get it right.'

That's as maybe but what we didn't bargain for was Diana refusing to drink the gloopy stuff. She would tip the tea away and make her own. She knew her own mind (well sort of) and no persuasion from us could make her see in the long run it was better for her, but I must admit the tea didn't look very appetising in fact it looked crap, even Diana could tell that. Her precious cuppa looked like thick brown poo. The Dementia had taken a bit of her reasoning away so it didn't matter what we said, she wanted her tea normal. Drinking a normal cuppa caused her at times to have choking fits. This was quite distressing for Diana and the kids and whoever witnessed it. At the beginning her swallow was ok, but with the Dementia she tended to shovel her food in and not take small sips or mouthfuls as Sian had explained. And she tended to slap your hand, if you tried to add the Thick and Easy to her drink. These were times when it became very frustrating. Lauren and Liam could get very impatient with their mother as they tried to follow everything that was told to them. They tried to do the best for their mother but with Dementia it was never going to be easy. It frustrated me and I didn't even live there so how did the two kids cope all day every day? If Diana hadn't had the Dementia then no problem, she would have followed the instructions to the tee. She followed the routine she remembered, she still tried to make Lauren's sandwiches for school which for Lauren must have been torture, as every day Lauren had a different concoction. Some days she gave Lauren one piece of bread with ham, no butter and no other slice on top, sort of like an open sandwich, other days, bread and butter and no filling at all. We laugh about it now but at the time poor Lauren must have dreaded opening her lunch box to find who knows what. Diana also still tried to make the dinner but it had to end when she dished up the kids half cooked sausages and hard mash potatoes. It then became Lauren's task to come home from school and start cooking. I knew this couldn't go on as Lauren couldn't possibly go to school, prepare their dinners and complete homework, and somewhere in between see her friends. Me and Mum would cook dinner for them a few times a week but we had to get something more permanent in place.

So we were introduced to the first lot of carers. Jack put this into place as soon as I told him about the sandwiches and uncooked food and the situation Lauren was now in. They were people that would come in to cook a dinner for the family; at first Lauren was reluctant, as she didn't want strangers in her home. I explained to her that it wasn't possible for me and Grandma to come every day, and cook not only our meals but theirs as well. I know she hated every minute of it, as most days it was a different person coming in. Lauren told me that she hated having to make conversations every day especially to a new face. They would ask Lauren questions about her mother, it wouldn't have been so bad but because of the new face every night it became a drag for Lauren. And Liam refused to stay downstairs and support her so this led to them arguing. I would then get a phone call from a tearful Lauren, then off I'd go and try and persuade Liam to stay downstairs with Lauren to give her a break. He promised me he would but he never did. And the annoying thing is every time a new face appeared Lauren also had to show them how the oven and the microwave worked. I told her to let them in and then go through to the sitting room to do her homework or watch telly but the carer would still seek her out to ask where certain things were and how they worked. So the poor girl couldn't get away from it. Diana didn't seem to mind these new faces coming in, she seemed to like the fact that she was being cooked for, but I had to tell whoever came that they needed to keep an eye on Diana as she shovelled her food in causing choking.

I was coming over quite a few times a week to help keep up with the housework and help Lauren with her homework. And the garden was becoming like a jungle, the grass was so overgrown you could hardly see the washing line. So we decided to tackle it, Liam mowed while me and Mum weeded, Diana sort of helped, it was a sort of automatic thing with her, we weeded she weeded, we dusted she dusted, we changed the bedding, she changed the bedding. There was one occasion when all four of us were working on the garden for the second time, it didn't seem to matter how many weeds we pulled out we didn't seem to make any headway. Diana has quite a big garden so it was a battle we probably wouldn't win. I pulled out weed after weed, well the ones I thought were weeds and there was Diana right next to me pulling at various tufts of whatever they were. In fact she seemed to be doing a better job than me; the whole time her face was completely expressionless. She was obviously copying me, she just pulled out a weed walked over to the bin threw it in, turned round and did the same again. It was like she had been programmed like a robot, it felt so strange as normally we would have all chatted nineteen to the dozen, Diana making tea and supplying loads of goodies to eat. She was always like that, anyone that visited would be offered tea and sandwiches or whatever she had in her home, and she always had plenty, and she was always very generous.

It wasn't long before we were all knackered but we were pleased with our efforts. Liam went to make the tea a role he took over from his mum. We sat on the patio chairs in the warm sun, having a break from our work that had made the smallest impact on the jungle before us. As I looked over at Diana it was funny but sad at the same time. She was leaning forward in her chair her arms on her knees, her head bent forward and there dribbling from her mouth was a long stream of thick saliva. What made it amusing was that she kept it trickling in the same spot for ages while she created a little pool in front of her feet. She sat engrossed in what she was doing, her little puddle growing larger and larger. This long stream of saliva just kept on flowing; she even moved her head round and round to make the puddle grow larger in size. She was totally oblivious to us sat there watching her, she didn't even move when Liam put the tea on the table, she just sat mesmerized as she continued to watch her puddle grow. This continued for quite a while until her concentration was broken when Liam noticed and said, 'Mum, what are you doing? That's gross.'

She just looked at him then wiped her mouth, picked up her tea and drank it, with the good old Thick and Easy in it.

At some point in the day Mum and I would have to leave and go home. I stayed as long as I could but I had two dogs that had probably done little piles if not then puddles. That's when Diana would usually get upset. She hated us leaving, she would fetch her coat and try to put it on but her arms were too weak to pull it on. It didn't matter to her what time it was, time meant nothing to her anymore. We would try to explain to her that we were needed at home and we would see her the next day and that she would be having her food soon, that usually persuaded her to stay, not always but mostly.

Running two homes was very tiring. I would tell Mum to go earlier as some days she looked exhausted. It always made me worry that her cancer was wearing her down and not old age. I know she liked to help because as she said, 'It takes my mind off my illness.'

I would get home just as Adam came in and then dish up his dinner, if I had made any that is! Or thrown something together literally. Sometimes I was so exhausted I would sit down and within seconds I was asleep on our settee.

Some days I felt a bit annoyed when he came in from work and said how tiring his day had been. 'You're tired? I'm knackered,' I would snap. 'You try running two homes.'

It wasn't his fault of course; it wasn't any one's fault. It was just a bad situation that needed all hands on deck for Diana's sake and for the children's sake.

Adam was always very sympathetic and then made me a cup of tea. I by then would feel very guilty as I knew he got tired driving the hundreds of miles he did for a water softener company; his medication also had a part to play.

I found I couldn't sleep very easily when I did go to bed, as I needed time to unwind and I also needed time to myself, so I would let everyone go to bed, then I would make a pile of sandwiches, turn on the movie channel and watch a film. It was the only time I knew the phone wouldn't ring unless of course there was a problem. I felt pretty safe and on my own which is what I craved some days, but of course by morning I was zombie-like for lack of sleep and a right misery, with a thumping headache.

But whatever I was feeling was nothing compared to my amazing niece and nephew who never once disturbed me at night even though some nights for them were hell.

One thing Jack encouraged me to do was to claim carer's allowance for myself as I was practically running Diana's home. This I did; I received £53.12 per week, I then split the money between the two children as they needed it more than I did. At last they had a bit of money to spend instead of having to count every single penny. This was their pocket money I told them as looking after their mother was a wonderful thing they were doing. They deserved every penny.

Chapter 12

We saw Prof Coles again in September. Jack and Claire were both there so that they could discuss Diana's case properly. Diana didn't take much notice of the conversation which I was glad about as Prof Coles didn't pull any punches. I told her that Diana had been rubbing her shoulder recently and crying with pain. Prof Coles examined her thoroughly. She said she wanted Diana to have an x-ray on it just to check she hadn't hurt herself in any way. We talked about the blasted saliva. Prof Coles said she would prescribe Diana Buccastem which may help stem the amount of saliva. I told her that Diana cried a lot and was sleeping badly and keeping the children from their own sleep, so she prescribed Mirtazapine. This was a mild anti-depressant but it would also help her to sleep better. She told us about energy drinks and foods that could help Diana get the right amount of supplements that she was missing in her diet, these could be supplied on prescription. The more I learnt about Motor Neurone the more I felt it difficult to be positive, it brought with it one problem after another.

The following week Lauren, Diana and myself took a taxi to the local hospital, to have her arm x-rayed. The waiting room was quiet so we weren't kept waiting long. It was decided I would accompany Diana into the changing room while Lauren waited with our belongings in the waiting room.

I couldn't help it, I let out a gasp as I helped remove Diana's clothing. Her body was so thin and her spine was so prominent, I didn't expect to see this. I felt tears well in my eyes, I felt so very sad that my once happy-go-lucky sister was now so ill and her body so emaciated. I quickly wiped away my tears so Diana wouldn't see as she would also cry. I just jollied her along as I always did.

It was while we were waiting for a taxi to go home that Diana suddenly started having a very bad choking fit. Her saliva had been getting worse, some days worse than others. It wasn't like having too much mucous in your throat, this was bucket loads of the stuff. Lauren kept rubbing her back while Diana tried to clear the damn stuff while also trying to breathe. I kept trying to reassure her, I felt any minute she would drown in the damn stuff. If the choking continued we would have to seek help back inside the hospital. God this disease was cruel. An ambulance had pulled up and saw what was happening. He came over with one of those paper bowler hat things that they use in hospitals if you are sick and gave us a load of tissue. Very kind but these two things weren't going to help. Luckily with Lauren's vigorous rubbing the choking stopped. Diana couldn't even sip water because that would go down the wrong way and make her choke even more. This disease just didn't play fair. When we got home I rang Claire and explained what had happened and how bad her saliva had become and that the choking was distressing for her. It was then suggested by Claire that Diana should be provided with the fantastic sucker machine with the yanker (long tube which narrowed with hole in the end) attached to it. Claire said she would arrange for one of the nurses to drop one off, then she would come to show us how to use it.

It was a brilliant machine. If Diana became very bubbly we would turn on the machine to clear away her excess saliva. This Diana found very comforting, she would point at it constantly for whoever was holding it at the time to put it in her mouth (whether needed or not). The tube or the yanker as it is called is placed into the person's mouth. Its suck is just about right to collect the excess fluid but not enough to get stuck on the patient's skin or tongue so no damage or hurt can come to the patient. The Buccastem didn't really make a lot of difference, not that I noticed anyway, but in your mind you want to believe it is working.

I think we all felt happier that the sucker machine was in the house as at night if Diana woke choking, which was incredibly frightening, Lauren or Liam would turn on the sucker machine and remove their mother's terrible secretion. I so admire the two of them on the nights that this happened and what they had to do to help their mother. Not once did they ever wake me but they dealt with it themselves. I always said if they needed me they should phone, which I know they would have if things got out of hand, but they always seemed to cope. Incredible young human beings!

Lauren was also missing a lot of school but it couldn't be helped. The girl needed her sleep and some nights she wasn't getting any.

The three of us me, Mum, and Diana continued to go to the shops every Monday. It was Mum's banking day and I would sort out any bills that needed paying for Diana. Her walking, by now was so much slower, but her determination to carry on as normal was phenomenal.

She liked being with us and so while she still could she was included in our shopping outings. Of course I couldn't spend every day with her as seeing her like she was, was gut wrenching. I needed a break in the week just to be able to think of other things in my life and sort out my own home. Also the friends I saw for a cup of tea and a chat recharged my batteries. These times made me forget a little of what was round the corner. I wasn't running away because my every thought was of Diana. Mum also needed rest as at eighty-two it was far too much for her, so she would come to Diana's a few times a week to help with various things like hanging out washing or putting away clothes that had been washed. I knew she liked to come and do something as Diana's illness had hit her hard. No mother expects to bury their child before them. I couldn't imagine how I'd cope if anything ever happened to my three sons. They give me strength and are wonderful sons and I am proud of them all, including Liam and Lauren. The boys also have lovely partners.

By now my oldest son had moved back home with his very pregnant wife Chloe. The baby was due in October. John was a bricklayer and the work was very scarce so money was tight and with a hefty mortgage to pay each month they felt that letting out their flat they could save money and then move back home after a year. I did say to John that I was worried about our jack russell and a baby in the house, but John said, 'I'm sure it will be ok, Mum'. Roddie had never been around children except my friend's four-year-old granddaughter. Roddie was ok at first but she would not leave him alone. He began to growl as she persisted in patting and pulling him around. I had no choice but to put him and Charlie our Heinz 57 rescue dog into our conservatory. Roddie is a little dog that likes peace and quiet and he loves the sun but children are a different matter; he just wasn't used to them. Kids always make for the cute little dog; it's natural as they are little themselves. Now if they had played with Charlie, he has a different temperament; a big softie, who would be good with kids. So I was a bit worried about bringing a baby into the house.

So in we all crammed. We managed to find a place for everything. My youngest James had agreed to give up his big bedroom so that John and Chloe had room to fit in all their bedroom furniture and have space for a crib when the baby came. My husband's work stuff, dummy water softeners paperwork etc. had to be piled into our bedroom, as not having a garage things were usually stored in our small spare room. This was now to be occupied by James.

We were a little overcrowded in my bedroom as several boxes were piled on top of each other against the window wall. It was a stretch to reach the window to open and close it. It didn't bother me as this was a blip compared to my sister's serious illness. Luckily I have a good relationship with Chloe; she's a girl that gets on really well with most people.

Chloe suffers with a mood disorder so having experienced depression herself she understood where I was coming from when my moods were up and down.

The worry I had was my own depression rearing its head again, so talking to Chloe really helped at such a difficult time in my life.

Chapter 13

I carried around this awful feeling of dread with me, I tried hard to lock those thoughts away but then the next time I saw Diana, it would all come flooding back as she looked a little different and walked a little slower. Her right hand had started to change in appearance, this I had seen before where the muscles start to weaken and the fingers start to roll towards the palm. I could see that was going to happen and soon. Her hair looked so dull and lifeless. At first she would let Lauren wash it as her hands were now too weak to manage anymore. The whole time Diana would cry then as soon as her head was wrapped in a towel she behaved as if nothing had happened. It was impossible for Lauren to cope with this on her own anymore so I helped her at the kitchen sink. I had said to Diana previously that day, 'Would you like me to wash your hair for you?'

With that she nodded vigorously, but as soon as we wet her hair she made loud groaning, crying noises (almost as if we were torturing her) and tried to push our hands away. It was a struggle to get out all the soap and it became a battle every time her hair needed washing. In fact Lauren and I left it a little longer every time, as we both hated upsetting her. She never minded her hair being dried though, as Lauren plonked her in front of the telly while she dried it. Diana just watched the carefully selected program good as gold.

On one morning I had a phone call from Lauren, she was crying. She told me Diana had got stuck in the bath and couldn't get out and Lauren couldn't lift her out. I could hear Diana crying in the background as Lauren explained what had happened. She told me she had to wake Liam to help get her out. Thank goodness Liam had already removed the bathroom lock; as Diana's hands got weaker she was struggling to pull back the bolt.

I phoned Jack right away to tell him what had happened. He told me he would phone Ridgeway and request a bath seat, so that she could step into the bath and then sit while she had a shower. This, when it came, Diana liked as Lauren helped her onto the seat and then showered her but Diana would smack out at Lauren if she got the water near her hair. Diana's smacks never hurt as her hands were far too weak to do any harm and it was her only way of communicating, that and pointing. Lauren had started helping her mother shower everyday as Diana was very wobbly trying to climb in and out of the bath; it had also frightened Diana getting stuck in the bath.

I so admired the way these two kids looked after their mother. Liam would talk to her almost child-like and Diana responded to this. Lauren would brush her mother's hair and then lay next to her in bed while they watched telly together. If they asked Diana for a cuddle she gave them one. How much was genuine affection I don't know, but she always seemed pleased to see them whenever they came in after going off out for a break themselves.

But they also argued a lot because of the awful situation they were in. No two days were the same, so over I'd go to sort out the problem or just listen then try my best to help. It might be that Diana needed a shower or they couldn't get her to take her medication or they were tired because Diana hadn't slept. I knew it was so frustrating for them as being with Diana twenty-four-seven was enough to push anyone to their limit.

At first it was ok to leave Diana on her own without carers as Liam was usually in, then Mum or I would call in to spend the afternoon with them both. But it soon became apparent that it wasn't safe if Liam went out and left her on her own. Not only because of Diana's excess saliva, (this was always worse when she drank or ate), but sometimes she would leave the house to walk to our mother's and leave the front door wide open. She also began to make black coffee and cheese sandwiches and take them to the summer house and leave them there. Well as soon as I was told black coffee I knew who they were for; her ex drank black coffee. It was so sad that she actually thought she saw him, or believed that he was in the garden somewhere. It is quite common for people with Dementia to see things. Shadows and reflections can become a person to a Dementia sufferer. The summerhouse was mostly glass and had many reflections.

After seeing the little boy in the garden I truly believed that she could see Sean in the garden, one of his favourite places to be.

One day during her illness and it only happened the once she wrote down 'Where is Sean gone?' She looked so dreadfully sad, I didn't know what to say to her. 'He's not here, Diana,' I said. I then immediately changed the subject and said, 'I know let's go to Mum's for a cup of tea,' and with that she had forgotten what she had written down. It never happened again.

As Diana's Dementia took hold it made her behaviour more erratic. She would open the blinds in the front room windows, then ten minutes later close them again only to open them as she walked back into the room again. She would make black coffee sometimes three times a day and take it to the summerhouse. She became cross if the children tried to stop her. She would turn lights on and off which made the children shout at her, this then made her cry because she didn't realise what she was doing wrong.

Evenings could be tiring for them as Diana would go into their rooms when they were trying to sleep and open up their curtains, turn on lights and then close the door and leave; this became part of her extraordinary routine.

It was now clear to me that Diana needed a lot more care; and the pressure needed taking away from Liam and Lauren. I was going over as much as I could but I had so much to do at my home, I was running myself ragged. And I was worried about Mum.

The two kids looked exhausted; they were getting more and more frustrated and tired from Diana's night time antics.

I contacted Jack and told him that Diana's behaviour was changing and we all now needed help, especially Liam and Lauren; they were not getting much sleep at night. It wasn't that Diana was a danger to the children as she loved being with them, but now she could be a danger to herself, (although eventually it wouldn't have been safe for any of them). What if she tried to cross over to me and just walked out in front of the cars? I had already told her not to come to me because it was too dangerous for her, I would come to her. Which she seemed to understand, as she hadn't yet turned up, but what about the future as her Dementia took hold?

Jack decided to call a few of the local care agencies. He would explain to them about Diana's needs as it wasn't only the Dementia but the dreadful Motor Neurone that needed to be considered. Was there an agency that could cope with both of these?

One week later we sat in Diana's front room. Jack had two ladies with him and the manager from the chosen agency itself. One lady was called Carol, the other Amanda. It was decided there and then that Carol would start the very next day. Rather than Carol turn up at Diana's we decided we would meet at our mum's house at eleven a.m., then I would walk back with Carol and Diana, I would then leave them together. We had to do it like that because Diana always turned up at our mum's early in the morning, sometimes even before mum had left her bed. No persuading Diana would make her arrive any later; she sometimes left the house before Lauren was ready to walk round with her. Lauren would then walk on to school. It became another of Diana's routines but incredibly tiring for our mum and for Lauren.

Carol's time to finish at Diana's was six p.m. That first day, as soon as Carol left to go home, Lauren phoned, telling me that as soon as Carol had gone Diana sobbed her eyes out and kept tapping Lauren on the arm and shaking her head. I knew this had been too much too soon, even though I tried to explain to Diana that the carers were there to help her and the children. She just shook her head with an awful fear in her eyes. Of course she was scared, I felt dreadful for her that it had come to this. I couldn't get through to her why she needed help. She held on to my arm with tears and a pleading look in her eyes. I could almost hear what she might have said to me.

'Please why are you allowing this to happen to me, Jan? I don't understand.'

I knew then the carers had to be introduced very gradually to Diana, maybe a couple of hours a few times a week. This was a very big thing for Diana, Liam and Lauren to get used to. I know I would have hated having strangers in my house so this had to be done very slowly.

It was agreed by Jack and myself that I would still come over a couple of times a week and then Carol and Amanda would come in for a few hours three times a week. Jack also suggested that we had some kind of door alarm fitted so that if Diana did leave the house without anyone knowing the alarm would alert them.

There had been one incident a few weeks before when Diana had gone missing. This is what finally decided us to have an alarm fitted. Liam had rung me concerned as Diana hadn't turned up at our mother's. I went across to the house as Liam was frantic with worry, her handbag had gone, so had her coat. As we were deciding what to do she came in the front door. We were both so relieved to see her, in her hand was a plastic shopping bag with a box of washing powder in it.

I felt like bursting into tears as it was so sad. Thinking about it now she so badly wanted to carry on as normal, or maybe there were days when the Dementia was better than others; her face still looked so expressionless, but she knew she needed washing powder. My sister was in there somewhere, some days more than others. And what had happened at the checkout, when the girl spoke to her and she didn't respond? I hate the thought that she was thinking how rude my sister was when she didn't reply to her.

When I went home I cried my eyes out as the realisation hit me I was losing my sister and one of my best friends.

The carers coming in less did have its hiccups. Diana would suddenly grab her coat and leave the house so poor Liam would have to go with her, whether it be to the shops or our mother's. He could only return home when his mother was ready or if we were all meeting at Diana's then she would happily return home.

Lauren wasn't keen on one of the carers. I found her pleasant enough but she was very quiet. It was decided that she wasn't suitable as Diana needed treating a certain way. Almost like a child she responded to a soft voice, cuddles and hand stroking, she also liked to be chatted to and she loved to hold your hand.

Amanda was Diana's carer sent from heaven, we were truly blessed when she came.

Liam and Lauren being young loved Amanda. She was in her thirties, full of fun, and wonderful with my sister. She had long curly hair, lovely blue eyes and a wonderful personality. She was very tactile with Diana and being an ex-hairdresser she could chatter away no problem.

Diana responded to Amanda straight away. She let her help her with anything and loved Amanda cuddling her. I noticed how good Amanda was with the whole family and she even called our mum, Grandma. She'd have a laugh with the kids, cook their dinners, clean house, whilst getting Diana to help. She had an amazing way with her, understanding my family's needs was to me, incredible. She fitted in and how! She spoke to Diana like a mother to a young daughter, she would stroke Diana's hand and talk to her about programmes they would watch together, she just had an amazing way about her. I knew it was safe to tell Jack to increase Amanda's hours.

By now we had a new girl to replace Carol. I think it was an age thing, the children liked the youngsters, after all it wasn't only Diana that had to get used to the new faces invading their lives. I had liked Carol but Amanda was so perfect for a situation like this it was going to be hard to find another Amanda!

Debbie started coming every Monday. She was in her twenties and again had great rapport with the kids and was great with Diana. On the days that the girls went home early or had half days I would go over.

Debbie unfortunately had to leave as she wanted to pursue another job, so Katherine joined the team. She was young and pretty and again had a lovely caring way about her. The kids liked her from the start and both her and Amanda loved to cook so Lauren would come in from school and have a meal waiting for her instead of cooking it herself.

Our friend Mary would still come to Diana's for our Tuesday get together; me, Mary, Diana, Amanda, Mum, Liam, Chloe and sometimes Lauren if she was home from school. This was becoming more frequent as some nights Diana hardly slept. We would sit and talk and laugh, Diana would watch the telly, usually her favourite programme, repeats of Come Dine With Me. She would turn and look at us from time to time and she would wave at us which was quite comical especially if you had been sat there a while. How much she took notice of our chatter I don't know, but we included her in our conversations, after all she was why we were all there, and I didn't know how much longer we would have her so I wanted everything just as it had always been; something we had always done and would continue to do even to this day.

Lauren usually fell asleep at some point as she was so tired from the lack of sleep from the night before.

Mary would arrive always on time and kiss Diana's thin cheeks, sit down and our little gathering was complete.

If you hadn't seen Diana for a while it was a shock at how she altered week by week. For me the change was gradual, as I spent so much time at the house, but if one of my sons or a neighbour hadn't seen her for a while their eyes said it all.

Her body was becoming so frail and thin as her eating became more difficult, her food had to be mashed, her choking was more frequent; her eyes looked wide and large in their sockets, and her cheeks hollow.

I remember sitting near to her, her on the chair, me on the settee, leaning across to hold her hand. This I think she found comfort in, these were the times when she was still and peaceful, not scuffling from room to room; they were rare but less tiring.

Another effect from Diana's constant dribbling was the stains that were appearing all over her carpets, and some of her furniture upstairs and downstairs. Her clothing also becoming stained as she refused to wear any protection over her clothes. When she ate – for example, chocolate mousse, it would end up all down the front of her clothing. As she was gradually losing control of her facial muscles it became harder for her to keep her mouth closed. And as she didn't sit still for very long the constant dribbling was also staining the rugs in the dining room and lounge. As much as we wiped away these stains more would appear. Of course her own natural saliva was acidic so white stains covered her clothing, even the washing powder had trouble removing them all.

We threw quite a few items of her clothing away, then I would get Adam to run me to Sainsbury's or Tesco to replace many tops and trousers.

We had to throw out her lounge rug as it was ruined. Mum tried once to scrub them away with a kitchen brush but she was getting nowhere fast. And Diana had to be changed frequently as the front of her neck and the front of her clothes were soaked and stained with food, juice and saliva. If she hadn't had Dementia I know she would have allowed us to use some kind of protection on her front, but she was having none of it. We tried to place a small hand towel under her chin, but she grunted and slung it to one side. I believe the washing machine went up to three times a day. The washing line was always full of washing when the weather was good, if not the tumble dryer constantly whirred round whilst we tried to keep up with the horrendous amount of washing.

As for the amount of kitchen roll she got through which was used to wipe her incessant saliva. I can't even begin to count how many rolls she got through in a week.

Most people that called in were now used to the sucker machine. Some days it wasn't needed much then other days it was needed frequently. Claire had shown the carers how to use it, although it wasn't part of their job because of the agency policies! That also included lifting Diana when she couldn't lift herself up from her chair. But they just used their common sense so if Diana struggled to get up the carers would help her. The reason behind the strict rules was to do with the carers injuring themselves whilst attempting such lifts but if Diana needed help then they helped her.

They didn't have much choice really considering the amount of times Diana got up and down.

I sometimes found it hard to look at Diana as it made my heart ache that she was so ill. She looked like a small child sat in her chair that seemed to dwarf her, so thin so frail, and I could not do a bloody thing to change it.

By now another carer had joined the team as coming in every day was too much for just two carers as Diana kept them on their toes. She spent a great deal of time walking about the house, she seemed to lose the capacity to relax, she stopped lying in bed but got up as soon as she woke up. She would go through to Lauren at any time of the morning, wake her up and indicate she wanted a shower. This for a teenager must have been so annoying as most teenagers at the weekend probably don't leave their beds until well after lunchtime. This also happened before Lauren left for school. She would often arrive late to school because she had to give her mother a shower, then dress her and give her breakfast, and her medication. But even though Lauren was rushed and tired she would do as her mother indicated. Looking back now how those two kids coped was a credit to them and the love they had for their mother.

Of course there were days when we were all at each other's throats. Weekends were the hardest as the kids wanted the weekends free of carers but they then argued because they both wanted to go out. It was usually poor Lauren that stayed in. At first it wasn't too bad as if her friends called she would take Diana to our mother's and leave her there while Lauren went out for a bit, but it was obvious that it was too much to expect Mum to cope with.

Diana would sit for a while with Mum then suddenly jump up, open Mum's door and leave to go home. This happened a lot and it was far too much for an eighty-two-year-old to rush after her sick daughter, especially as Mum was having treatment herself.

So I would then spend some Saturdays sat in with Diana in the day so that Lauren could have a break, then they both came to me every Saturday evening as it gave Lauren someone to chat to and different walls to look at, and company as Lauren found being at home very depressing and very quiet if Liam was out. I had tried hard to persuade Liam that if he went out one day he should stay in the next so Lauren could go out. But Liam resented staying in; he is so young in his ways so staying in to him was like a punishment regardless of how his sister was feeling.

This is when the arguments would start. And even if we did get him to agree that the following weekend he would stay in, he would soon forget (deliberately) about it and go out causing yet more tension.

Sian the speech therapist was coming in regularly now, as Diana's swallowing needed checking more frequently. It was becoming difficult for Sian to make Diana understand that the best way to swallow was to keep her head back and her chin up as she swallowed, this helped the food go down easier. Diana would watch as Sian demonstrated. 'Now you try, Diana'.

But Diana just couldn't grasp what was being requested of her and would do it her own way and move her head towards the spoon in her hand, and then shovel its contents in. It was the Dementia that made it impossible for Diana to understand what was required of her. It was my idea that Diana should use a teaspoon so that she could only load her mouth with a certain amount of food, which was obviously safer for her. She couldn't shovel it in then as the spoon only held a small amount of food. Also Sian wanted the carers to sit with Diana at mealtimes now to prevent her from putting in another mouthful until she had finished the last one. 'Hold her arm down until her mouth is empty,' Sian instructed.

Sian also brought with her a speech board, it had pictures on it. For example, if Diana wanted a cup of tea she could push the little panel with the cup and saucer picture, it would say, 'I would like a cup of tea.' It had various things Diana could request and quite good fun but again the Dementia prevented her from understanding its usefulness. She would just push one panel after the other, 'I would like a cup of tea, I am tired, I want to go to bed, I want to go out.' To Diana it was more fun than practical. 'I'll leave it here. Perhaps Diana will get used to using it on her own,' Sian announced.

I knew better. As soon as Sian had gone Diana took it upstairs and pushed it under her bed which indicated she didn't want it and she wouldn't use it. Things Diana didn't want were shoved in drawers or under her bed. I had to instruct Lauren that when the postman came she should take the letters before her mother got to them so that she couldn't hide them away before I could deal with them. As I was dealing with everything connected to the house I needed to see any post that arrived.

Everything out of the ordinary was the Dementia's fault. Her continuous walking around the house, upstairs then back down, into the kitchen, into the loo, back through to the lounge, open the fridge, look in, grab a yogurt, leave fridge door open, grab a spoon leave drawer open, eat it, get back to kitchen, grab another, during all this someone had to follow her because she was so unsteady on her feet.

There were however a few telly programmes that kept her seated like, *Come Dine With Me*, and *How Clean is Your House?* and *Wild at Heart*. These programmes she was completely focused on.

On restless days which now were becoming more frequent, she would open and close the blinds a few times going from one room to the next. She switched on lights then turned them off again. This she repeated many times. She would try to open the front door which we now kept locked for her safety, she would become agitated and push Lauren pointing to the door. She wanted Lauren to find the well hidden key and unlock it. It didn't matter what time of the day or night it was, if Diana got it into her head she wanted to go out it was very difficult to distract her or reason with her. We also found the freezer in the garage switched off. No one knew when she had done it, and it could only have been Diana, so everything had to be thrown away. A few bits we cooked and re-freezed. She then had to be watched like a hawk; all this was very tiring. Due to lack of money there was no contents insurance so the ruined food couldn't be claimed for.

I asked the kids to regularly check in case the freezer had been switched off as there wasn't the money to keep replacing lost food.

She didn't like any of her possessions moved. I once moved one of her lamps to give more light in the lounge, she then moved it straight back. All this I attributed to her Dementia.

I do believe, however, the Dementia saved her from a very distressing and frightening time when it came to her Motor Neurone. I can't think of anything worse than losing the ability to swallow. I was frightened for her every day of her life. Maybe this was God's act of kindness; they say God only gives you what you can cope with. Diana would never have coped with Motor Neurone. It was a blessing that she never knew that she would never see her children again and that she didn't have long to live. In a way the Dementia saved us as well as I would have hated seeing my sister so distressed and frightened every day, and not being able to reassure her, as for God's sake, what reassurance could I have given her? Knowing this unrelenting illness would take her away from her family and us would have destroyed all her faith in God. She was in her own little bubble and things said one minute to her were forgotten the next.

There were some days I just couldn't see her. I felt so guilty at avoiding seeing her but it gave me time to recharge my batteries and cope with my own feelings. I always tried to keep myself upbeat especially for Liam and Lauren; their lives were depressing enough without their aunty breaking into floods of tears every five minutes. And they relied on me to make the right decisions for their mother and themselves.

I would joke around with them, which would make them laugh then the atmosphere would change for a bit. Amanda and Katherine were much the same; happy good-natured people, they brought the normality back into their lives. Lauren would come in from school and dinner was waiting for her, that hadn't happened for a while! They became someone she could talk to and share her day at school with, just as she used to with her mother. Liam liked their company and he was free in the day to go out if he wanted to. They became part of the family and were very important to all of us.

Both Amanda and Katherine would take Diana out in their cars. This she loved; she would get her coat and go straight to the front door not even waiting for windows to be closed or doors locked. She was like an impatient child waiting for a treat. If Lauren was home she would go with them, Liam also if he wasn't meeting friends. Amanda would take them into Newbury to look around the shops then stop somewhere for a drink and cake. At the beginning Diana could manage a soft cake and tea, but eventually it became impossible to take her for food as her swallowing became worse. Everywhere Diana was taken, which wasn't too far, reams of tissue had to go with her because of her dribbling.

By now Diana's arm and hand were useless. Her hand now remained in a permanent claw shape bent towards her wrist and her fingers looked tight and swollen.

She would cry and hold her shoulder. It was obvious she was in quite a lot of pain so I contacted her doctor and she put out a prescription for Traxem gel to try and ease the pain.

Amanda would also massage Diana's poor hand when she applied the gel. This seemed to ease her pain and it was obvious it relaxed her, as she never went walkabout during these sessions.

It was the changes in her that made it so hard for us all, the constant reminder that her body was in decline and there was no going back.

Mum also suggested a hot water bottle with a fluffy cover on it. Diana actually sat still when we gave her a hot water bottle, this also must have helped the pain. All these things I had to remember so that I could tell Professor Coles and I had many questions I wanted to ask.

Prof Coles' nurse Claire came in quite regularly to see Diana. She became a fantastic lifeline as problems began to rear their head. It was decided that Prof Coles would visit Diana at home at her next visit, after being told about Diana's massive choking fit outside the hospital.

The dreaded tissue was also causing problems, a bin had been placed by Diana's chair so that the tissue, (it was actually kitchen roll as it was so absorbent) could be thrown away but at night Diana would throw the stuff down the toilet. This then led to the drains blocking and the downstairs loo overflowing. I then had to ask the next door neighbour if he could use his drain rods to unblock the loos and the drains, three to four times we had to request his help in the freezing cold to unblock the offending tissue before it blocked the drains in the house the other side of Diana's. In the end we had no choice but to use toilet tissue instead for Diana's dribbling. It wasn't as good but we couldn't make Diana understand not to throw the kitchen roll in the loo.

We also had to make the decision that it was now too much for Diana to walk too far, that included to our mother's. Instead Diana could be taken out by car and wander slowly around the shops as this she always enjoyed, linking arms with whoever was on the trip with her. And instead of Diana and Lauren coming to my home every Saturday night to watch programmes we would go over to them. As not being able to take much food she was very weak, she was also very unsteady on her feet. She fell asleep quite a bit in the day and early evening. So us joining them we could get Diana into her pyjamas and make her more comfortable, then if she did fall asleep while we were there it didn't matter.

I had spoken to Jack about Diana's chairs and that they were now too difficult for Diana to get out of, unless she had help. It was difficult to lift her as being so thin it hurt her if held under her arm so she had to be held around the waist and eased up which was a strain on the person's back doing the helping.

Liam didn't find it too difficult; he is quite strong so if he was around it was helpful.

So it was decided that she be measured for a special chair, a recliner that could lift her up and lower her down. Her measurements had to be precise, her length from knees to her back when sat, also her height, and her length from head to lower back, then from her bent knees to her feet. I was pleased that so much care was taken over her measurements to ensure her comfort and she seemed to enjoy the attention.

While we were waiting for the chair to arrive we had to lose a chair to accommodate the new recliner. The chair we needed to move was crammed into the extension next to another small settee at the end of the room. It was a bit cluttered but at least we could keep the chair until it was needed again. It didn't matter though as Diana's needs were greater so everything that could be done we did. Anything to make her life a little easier. I already had the kettle changed to one that had a special safety pourer attached to it. Also stair gates were fitted top and bottom so that Diana didn't tumble down the stairs. If she wanted to go upstairs she had to wait until it was opened for her then she could be accompanied upstairs or downstairs as her legs were extremely weak especially climbing stairs.

It was also decided that the front door be kept locked at all times as many a time she went off, without us knowing. It was becoming unsafe for her to go anywhere unaided.

The house also had to be kept hot day and night, as being so thin Diana felt constantly cold, not very comfortable for anyone else but in this case that didn't matter. By the time visitors left they had a definite red tinge to their cheeks.

All appointments that concerned Diana were held at her home. One person Diana took to right away was a guy called Mark. He came from Newbury hospital from the mental health team. It had been decided that Diana take a drug that would help try and change the chemicals in the brain. It is an antipsychotic, the drug in question was called Risperdal. It is not usually used on people that have Dementia but after reading up on it and although it was never discussed I assume it was because my sister was seeing things and she was very agitated. It was orodispersible, as she could not swallow tablets. Mark would call round to check how Diana was getting on with these drugs and that she wasn't suffering any side effects, as I believe it had quite a few. If Diana knew he was coming, it's really strange but she always wanted clean clothes on for his visit and not her messy ones that she wore until they were messy. Don't get me wrong Diana was changed about three or four times a day and the washing machine went continuously. She would point to go upstairs and open her chest of drawers and hand over to whoever had accompanied her the clean clothes she wanted to wear. We all thought it was so sweet that she wanted to look nice when he came and she liked to hold his hand. Diana obviously liked and trusted him, hence the clean clothes and the hand holding. (I must admit he did have quite a sexy voice.) How much Risperdal helped her I have no idea but it made you feel that it might make her quality of life better, at least she wasn't seeing things anymore. Although she wouldn't have been able to tell us any more if she did see things, she wasn't able to communicate, only pointing or shaking her head.

Her arm was still playing her up as she would cry at me and indicate her shoulder hurt by pointing and holding it while she cried. The Traxem gel wasn't enough now. I called Claire who spoke to Prof Coles who in turn contacted Diana's doctor. Prof Coles had decided that Diana could have a pain patch. She requested that her doctor come to see us to explain that there were a few side effects, one being constipation (I don't remember the others). I hated seeing Diana cry in pain with her poor arm, it was impossible to give her any painkillers orally as her swallowing was so bad. 'I want her to be pain free,' I told the doctor.

She then told me to call if Diana did suffer with constipation as things could be done to help her.

It took a couple of days after the patch was applied until Diana stopped holding and crying about her arm, but I found myself asking Lauren, 'Has your mum pooed today?'

'I don't know,' came the reply, 'I don't stay in the loo with her, you're gross, Aunty Jan.'

We both laughed when I suggested that Lauren should go in after her mum had been to the loo and sniff! Diana always shuffled out of the toilet with her underwear round her ankles before Lauren got there to help her re-dress. The Dementia had taken away her sense of privacy and inhibitions. It didn't matter who helped her as long as her clothes were pulled up.

If there were males in the house e.g. my hubby or Liam, we had to wait outside the loo door so that you could dress her in private before she scurried out in front of them.

I called it poo watch, (poor Lauren being the main watcher). I hated the idea of her being constipated and unable to tell us if she was uncomfortable. We always cheered when she had been; even Diana seemed to know why we cheered. It was all done in a kind and jovial way and not in any way to disrespect her, I would never do that to her. I tried to take the seriousness out of things and situations that happened and make them seem less important. That was for the children's sake more than anything, as this disease was scary enough without all the problems that could arise.

I also at some point had to decide when to tell Liam and Lauren that their mother would not survive this. Liam knew his mother was ill and Lauren was with us when the consultant said, 'No treatment, no cure,' but I knew Lauren didn't realise just how serious this really was.

I knew I couldn't leave it too long as she was deteriorating day by day.

It would be the most difficult thing in my life that I had to do, there was never going to be a right time, so at present I just left things as they were.

Of course the inevitable happened and Diana did suffer with constipation, so once again another treatment had to be decided. This time it was to be a suppository and the district nurse would come in every other day to insert it, this we hoped would keep things moving so to speak.

By now Diana was having Ensure drinks. This was a supplementary food, it came in various flavours. There were also Ensure yogurts; these Diana seemed to manage quite well. Poor girl must have been so hungry, as all her food had to be blended now, she would start to eat and then at some point have a choke, then she would push the food away.

This was a continuing cycle. I knew that people with Motor Neurone usually end up having a feeding tube; it had been mentioned once by Sian. Diana's reaction to this was quite bad she shook her head and stared at me wide eyed like a frightened child and frantically tapped my arm. She was trying to tell me that she didn't want the feeding tube.

It was weird that there were things she did understand and others she had no notion of.

It wasn't mentioned again until Prof Coles next saw Diana.

Our lives continued on with one problem after the next. As they appeared they were dealt with, it became a familiar pattern, it was like we were all in robot mode, and everything seemed so unreal. We had been presented with a nightmare to live in, and as we walked towards the door to get away, the door moved further and further away from us. Would I wake up and realise it was just a bad dream? But every morning I woke it hit me the nightmare was still here.

Liam's and Lauren's lives were the biggest nightmare as it was twenty-four-seven for them. Sean will never know how much they had to cope with, and how incredibly brave they were looking after their sick mother.

Chapter 14

My phone without fail rang every morning, even before I had the energy to crawl from my warm comfortable bed; the calls were mostly connected with Diana. I felt like a doctor, nurse, secretary, psychiatrist, wife, mother, daughter, aunty, telephonist, carer. All these words sat there on my shoulders and as they applied I went into that mode, it became automatic. I had stopped feeling sorry for myself the day Diana was diagnosed. Yeah, I still moaned mainly to my friends; it was a relief to share how I felt with them. I was a right misery to be with and definitely no fun. It was just off loading, freeing up my over loaded brain ready for the next problem.

It is difficult to stay upbeat when you live with so much negativity going on; it's going to drag you down with it. So the support Diana had was invaluable. Without it we would have sunk months ago. They were the real doctors, nurses, carers, etc. I just went on the same path using my instinct and common sense. Knowing my sister so well I knew how she would want things done, and how Liam and Lauren should be looked after, they would always have been Diana's main priority.

I know Lauren loves to clothes shop, she has her favourite T.V. programmes, T.O.W.I.E and Glee being her favourites, she hates germs, she can't bare ripping paper, or touching cotton wool, sick makes her sick! She loves jewellery and handbags and owns many, she prefers to wear trousers and not dresses, she's a giggler, she hates washing up, she loves Ant and Dec, she is very close to her brother, and she loved her mum more than anything.

Liam loves music especially dance, he's a very talented D.J., he has become very good at ten pin bowling and usually wins, he loves red sauce, gallons of the stuff and subways, he loves his bed and his computer, he loves his X-box, he has an infectious dirty laugh, his mates are very important to him, he needs encouragement to give him confidence, he's become very good with the washing machine, which is then taken straight to the tumble drier, even on hot days! (Oh dear the electricity!) He doesn't mind food shopping for anyone, he too hates washing up, he desperately wants a job that he can manage, and that pays him enough to survive on as he is now the main bill payer, he is very close to his sister, and he also loved his mum more than anything. They are both so very young to have lost her from their lives. I feel sad and angry that Diana isn't here anymore to guide them as mothers do and to spend time with them as I do now.

I will never understand why this should happen to them. If anyone needed a mother it is Liam, I don't mean Lauren doesn't, but she is mature for her age and is going from strength to strength, but Liam with his disabilities really needed Diana reassuring and pushing him along as she always did. It is a cruel world we live in and what those two were dealt sucks! If your life is mapped out for you then theirs wasn't a fair hand. Life is what you make it, (I don't think so!) what a crap start they have had.

My part in all this? Be there when they need me; advise as I think Diana would; deal with problems as they arise; encourage, support, nurture; keep an eye on Liam's spending (he's not too good at budgeting, it's part of his disability). Make birthdays, Easter, and Christmas fun, make sure they are at all our family gatherings and more importantly always talk about Diana. She will stay in our hearts forever.

Chapter 15

Every Friday Adam and I would take Mum, Diana and Lauren food shopping to Lidl. Our car would heave under the weight of all the shopping. As Diana deteriorated it became too much for her so it was decided that I would go with a list and do their shopping for them. This at least left space on the back seat beside mum. Adam's car was always full up with his endless work gear, boxes of leaflets and dummy water softener display units, so before we even left to go shopping he had to unload quite a bit just to get us all in.

Sometimes Lauren could sneak out while Diana stayed with her carer. She just wanted to get out of the house for an hour or so. When we returned Adam and I would help Lauren unpack the shopping. I was also then returning back to their house Friday evenings to keep them company as the carer left at eight. We watched *Coronation Stree*t and *Eastenders*, these programmes Diana liked, and it was nice for Lauren to have someone to talk to as Liam usually went out with his mates.

On one particular Friday evening as we returned from shopping I noticed Diana's breathing seemed deeper and it sounded raspy, I could see her chest rising quicker and higher than normal. I decided to ring our after hours doctors to request a home visit. As I put the phone down, Diana was there behind me, she looked worse and blue around her mouth, her face looked clammy and her skin glistened, her breathing was more laboured, she also looked extremely frightened. So I phoned back the same number as I knew you can wait for ages until a doctor comes, this was now more urgent. They told me to ring an ambulance, which I did right away. Diana became agitated and breathed heavier, her eyes wide with fear, as soon as she heard me requesting an ambulance. I held her hand and tried to explain that she needed to be seen, I sat her down, Lauren sat with her holding her hand and stroking it. 'It's ok, Mum, you'll be fine.' I felt very fearful, was this the end already? Before I even had time to prepare them both for losing their precious mother. I prayed silently that it wasn't.

I couldn't and still can't believe everything that was happening to us as a family. My sister didn't deserve any of this.

Minutes later the ambulance pulled up. They checked her thoroughly, but she refused to wear the oxygen mask one of the crew tried to place on her face. She kept pushing it away, all the time she looked at me with wide and fearful eyes. If she could have spoken I know she would have said, 'Jan, help me, I am so scared.'

That's exactly what her eyes were saying to me; she looked at me the whole time. I wanted to smash the Motor Neurone out of her to crush it as it was crushing her. It is a bloody Bastard of a Disease. I hated it, despised it and loathed it and I wouldn't wish it on my worst enemy.

As I was talking to the ambulance crew the doctor I had requested also turned up. It was a young lady doctor. She checked Diana over as the paramedic had. 'Diana has a chest infection,' she told us. 'I can leave you penicillin or she can be seen in hospital.'

There was no question as to our choice. Her swallowing was poor, it would be impossible to try and give her medicine as most of it would end up down her clothing. And she looked far too ill to be treated at home.

Her colour was a bluish grey and her skin looked transparent, I could see how ill she was, leaving her penicillin wasn't an option.

It had to be hospital. Lauren and Liam looked very frightened; this was the first time we had ever called an ambulance. Many doctors, yes, but not an ambulance. I told them both that in hospital they could treat their mother and make her more comfortable and get the antibiotics into her so much easier than we ever could.

Lauren and I went upstairs and grabbed a few items of clothing, her wash things and her current medication.

We put on her coat, which now swamped her small frame. As we walked into the cold night air I shivered more from fear

I think than cold. Diana's house was kept very warm day and night so the cold would definitely affect Diana. It was like walking from a greenhouse into a freezer, her tiny thin body got so cold these days. I could see the ambulance had caused quite a stir with the neighbours, these weren't your nosy neighbours they were concerned ones and would have all helped if asked.

I could also see Diana's neighbour Rita opposite watching from her window. She always left her curtains open so that she could keep an eye on them and the house since they had been left on their own. It was great that Rita kept an eye on the house in case there were any unwanted visitors as sometimes there were. And on the odd evening she came to spend time with them as the evenings in for Liam and Lauren were monotonous and very hard work. Once when I was on holiday Lauren was feeling really poorly it was Rita that took her and my mum down to the doctors and waited to bring them home again. She has been brilliant and so have a few of the other neighbours, bringing food and visiting Diana and offering their services. But Rita has been the best and still is. It felt safe that they were living in a small secure no through road. I never worried when I went home, any of the neighbours would help in a crisis.

The paramedic led Diana to the ambulance steps; he helped her up with Lauren right behind. Adam and I got into our car to follow, as I looked over there was Diana climbing back down the steps and heading for our car. She did not want to go in the ambulance; and no persuading would encourage her back into it. She opened our back door and slid herself in.

'We can't force your sister into the ambulance. It's ok if she rides with you,' the paramedic told us.

'What if she takes a turn for the worse?' I asked.

'Just phone us and we will come to you.'

I wasn't very happy about it but we had no choice.

So off we went. I felt very anxious with her sat in the back with Lauren, it was quite a ride to The Royal Berks Hospital and her breathing was heavy and laboured. We couldn't go through traffic lights like an ambulance could. I felt a bit let down by them, but I suppose they couldn't use force. And what if she collapsed or worse stopped breathing? I felt shaky and very nervous again. I could see in the mirror her wide, frightened eyes that shone in the dark. Lauren clutching her hand to reassure her.

And sod's law we were caught by every bloody traffic light that we came to. Luckily it wasn't too busy on the roads as by now it was nine p.m.

Adam drove us straight to casualty; he then went to find a parking space.

There was another ambulance outside casualty; I grabbed one of the wheelchairs and sat Diana in it, I called to a lady paramedic who was getting out from the said ambulance, I explained how ill Diana was. Thank goodness she took us straight through the back entrance. I gave a nurse at the desk the letter from the doctor who had originally seen Diana.

We were taken straight to an empty cubicle, we helped Diana onto the bed. She was so fragile it was too much for her to attempt to climb up herself, it was difficult to make her comfortable as I was afraid of hurting her.

We made her as comfortable as we could but we didn't have the strength to move her without hurting her painfully thin arms and legs, between Lauren and I her body was a dead weight.

It was then half an hour before a nurse came. She apologised and told us it was very busy that night. She put an oxygen mask onto Diana's face, Diana immediately smacked it away, which shocked the nurse. I explained that Diana had Dementia and basically she was frightened because she didn't understand what was happening to her.

So Lauren held the mask to the side of Diana's face, so that it wasn't covering her mouth and nose, this she didn't object to. The nurse also took some blood and put a clip thing on her finger I think this measures your oxygen input. She told us the doctor would be round as soon as he had seen other patients in front of Diana.

I prayed there weren't many, but I could tell by the amount of noise and hustle and bustle it was very, very busy. One hour went by, then two. I stopped the nurse as she went by. 'How much longer now?'

'Sorry the doctor shouldn't be much longer, it's just so busy tonight.'

I felt like shouting, 'For fuck's sake my sister is seriously ill. Leave all the bloody drunks in their vomit!' (There were a few in that night.) But I didn't, I would have been thrown out.

By now I could see Diana was very uncomfortable sat upright and still on the hospital bed. She wasn't strong enough to move herself into a more comfortable position, as her right arm now was completely useless. Sitting in the same position for so long was making Diana's legs and backside numb.

I could tell as she kept fidgeting. 'We need to get your mum into a chair,' I told Lauren. I looked out from behind our curtain, there opposite in another cubicle was a very comfortable looking soft chair. The people who had occupied it previously had now gone.

He had been a drunk and gone once he had sobered up a bit and been able to walk.

Lauren without any prompting from me walked straight across and carried the chair back for her mother. Between us we helped Diana down from the bed onto the chair making sure we didn't loosen any of her wires.

She looked more comfortable and seemed less agitated although the big chair swamped her small pathetic frame.

'I'll go and see Adam in the waiting room, as he'll wonder what has happened to us. If the doctor comes say where I have gone,' I instructed Lauren.

The casualty waiting room was packed; it had to be as the cubicles I left behind were all full. There were many people like Adam waiting for loved ones or waiting to be seen.

There he was sitting between two women, his elbows on his knees and his head drooping towards his, I can only say his privates, fast asleep. It looked a very precarious and uncomfortable way to sleep I called him but he didn't wake so I signalled to one of the women who I could see looked most amused that anyone could fall asleep in such a position. She tapped his shoulder; he jumped up which made the woman jump. He walked over to me with dribble on his chin. Typical Adam he could sleep anywhere, he would probably find a bed of nails comfortable, nothing stops him sleeping. 'We're still waiting for a doctor,' I told him.

'Ok, girl,' (my pet name), came his sleepy reply.

Thank God he was such a patient person, and knowing what casualty can be like he knew we might be ages. 'No problem I'll get myself a drink,' and back he went to his seat.

Finally at three a.m. a very tall well-spoken African doctor came into our cubicle. I noticed how tired he looked; it had obviously been a very long shift for him. He apologised for our long wait, then asked question after question. Diana sat in her chair she looked so tired poor thing, I found it hard not to be abrupt with him at our long wait, but it wouldn't make things different if I had. So we stood there answering his questions as best we could.

As soon as he listened to Diana's chest he ordered a chest X-ray straight away. A porter came almost immediately and collected Diana; Lauren and I followed behind. We went into the corridor, the X-ray room was right opposite from casualty. We waited outside, both of us yawning setting the other off.

At last Diana was being dealt with but it was so difficult to be calm when someone you love is so very ill.

Diana had only been back in the cubicle for a matter of seconds when a male nurse rushed in and injected her with I can only assume were antibiotics.

Diana, we were told had pneumonia.

All this time she had waited and now finally everyone was rushing here and there; she was found a bed immediately on a ward and taken there straight away by wheelchair.

It was the C.D.U., which stands for Clinical Decision Unit. As soon as she saw the ward and a bed she became agitated and tried to get out of her wheelchair. I took hold of her hand to try and reassure her but she kept shaking her head and trying to pull out her wires that were in her arms. I knew the only thing to do was to leave as she would never settle with Lauren or me there. Already patients were waking up with the noise.

The nurse did say we could stay with her but Lauren was so tired and so was I, and I really did not have the energy to chase Diana around a ward where other patients were trying to sleep.

It, as it turned out, was the best thing to do; as soon as we had left the ward the nurses sat Diana in a chair at the nurse's station so that she had company. Diana had refused to get in bed and kept trying to find the door to get out and follow us. So sitting her with them for a while calmed her down. She was much better when we weren't around.

If we had stayed we would have played cat and mouse all night, I knew I had made the right decision.

On the way home the streetlights annoyed me they were so bright, as my eyes ached for sleep and felt gritty because of the amount of time I had been wearing my contact lenses. I pulled down the sun screen to block the annoying lights, I could see in the mirror Lauren was nearly asleep. I think we both knew Diana was in good hands, we had done the right thing I felt sure of it, and we would visit her the next day.

As soon as I got home I rang the ward to check on her.

She was ok I was told; once she realised we had gone she was calmer and more responsive to the nurses' requests. They had put a drip in her arm with antibiotics and one because she was very dehydrated. They had managed to coax her into bed and a nurse was feeding her a cup of tea with Thick and Easy in it.

I can't tell you how relieved I was. I felt guilty leaving her there but I had not been home since five p.m. that previous day and Adam had work in the morning. He was shattered as he had been up since six a.m. the previous day.

His precarious sleep in the waiting room didn't count!!

I had to consider everyone's needs and I knew the hospital would do their best to make Diana well again or as well as they could considering her illness.

Liam and Lauren also had a good undisturbed night's sleep, which they hadn't had for a very long time.

But as usual I found it hard to sleep, I was mentally exhausted and extremely worried, but sleep wouldn't come as so many thoughts were running through my aching head, so I turned on our telly in the bedroom and watched some daft late film. I can't even remember what it was about because it was pretty awful. I must have fallen asleep with it on as I woke wondering why my bedroom was so bright, and now I was bloody well awake again. I hated it when morning came. It was safe in bed. The only trouble with bed is I tend to think of everything and everyone; all problems are mulled over until your head aches, the more I tried not to think the more I thought. I believe there should be some device that makes you switch off and relax and sleep a restful sleep as soon as your body hits the mattress. How many times had I rehearsed in my head a speech that I was going to use in an important phone call the next day? Too many bloody times that's how many, or what I was going to write in a letter or an email in the morning? Or what did I need to request from the doctor the following morning? On and on into the early hours, think, think, think. Shame you can't remove your brain at night, lay it next to you on your pillow and zonk; a good night's kip!!

So I read or watched telly or a DVD until I couldn't keep my eyes open anymore. I had to occupy my brain another way, as sleep would never come.

As soon as it was a respectable time I phoned the C.D.U. to ask after Diana. She'd had a good night and she slept for a bit the nurse told me on the other end of the phone.

'I will be in to see her later,' I told the nurse.

Lauren did not want to come with us, she had found the night before extremely difficult.

Deep down these episodes with Diana frightened them both. This was their precious mother, sometimes they needed time away to be normal and try and forget what was happening to her and to them. And they must have missed her dreadfully; the strong well Mum that took care of everything in their lives.

So it was agreed that Adam and I go in. I was actually dreading it as I knew Diana would think we were there to take her home. I was right. As soon as she saw me she started to cry; she held out her arms to me like a child to its mother. This was going to be very difficult.

I was so shocked by her appearance, her skin looked almost transparent, her face looked thin and skeletal, her eyes protruded from their sockets. There was a greyish tint to her skin, she looked very old and frail today, in the daylight I could see just how ill she really was. If I had pinched her skin, it would have stayed in that position. At that moment I thought to myself my sister didn't have very long to live, this was going to be her end, here in this crowded ward. She looked so awful. I wanted to cry but I couldn't.

My heart was beating rapidly as I tried to keep calm, I felt so scared as I had not experienced someone so close to death before.

I had to keep calm, I could not get upset in front of her, she picked up so easily on everyone's mood. Anyone acted differently she knew. So I took a deep breath and sat down next to her on her bed, I felt sure she would hear my heart thumping in my chest. I'm ashamed to say I didn't cuddle her as I knew this would make her cry and I hated her being upset. The whole time she not once took her eyes from my face, her large frightened lovely green eyes that looked too big for her bony sockets. I could almost hear her mind ticking over waiting for me to say it was time to leave, and for me to pack up her belongings and take her home. At that very moment I wanted to be anywhere but here. She had wires fed into her arm as they pumped in antibiotics and fluids. She had to stay still because these pumps were plugged into sockets in the wall above her bed, she kept pulling at them to remove them from her arm; she really believed I would be taking her home with me. It was difficult to distract her from doing this. I tried to chatter on but her eyes bored into me, she was pleading with me through her eyes and looked piercingly straight into mine. I had to look away; I felt guilty and such a cow, and I felt frustration that I couldn't make her understand that she wasn't being punished and that when she was better she could come home. I took her thin hand into mine stroking it, and tried to explain why she was there, and that I wasn't being cruel.

'They will make you so much better, Diana.'

But she heard none of it, her Dementia took away all reasoning, it took away her understanding, and it had taken her away.

Other patients in the ward had magazines or crossword books and the daily paper, all of these were pointless for Diana. Above her bed it read Nil by mouth.

(They had decided not to give her anything else by mouth until her swallowing had been checked.)

Oh, God, I thought, she must be so thirsty, her mouth must be so dry. I brushed a tear from my cheek, I couldn't, mustn't get upset.

I knew we would have to leave soon as I had to let out my feelings that were over whelming me. I knew I would cry any minute. I could feel it welling up inside me.

We stayed for about an hour which was long enough, the whole time she held my hand as if her life depended on it, now was the hard bit, trying to leave.

Adam went to fetch a nurse to sit with her to prevent her from pulling the plugs out of their sockets on the wall and the wires from her arm, as I knew she would try to follow us.

It was exactly what she tried to do; as I looked back her poor pale thin face was contorted with the look of sheer terror; her sister had left her again. She was crying making awful groaning noises, she looked at me pleadingly. She wanted to come with us. The nurse was having trouble holding on to her. She wanted to be back in the safe place where everything was familiar to her; I can only imagine what she felt as we walked away. My frightened, terribly sick, much loved sister.

Back in the car I sobbed my eyes out. Life was shit; Motor Neurone was shit. As we drove away I honestly believed my sister didn't have much longer with us.

I made a tearful phone call to our mum and said how difficult it had been for us. I was honest with her, I told her I really believed Diana wouldn't last the week. I told her that we should all go in next time, as it was too difficult visiting on our own. I needed support from other members of my family to get through this myself.

At that moment it suddenly hit me my sister was actually going to die, and it hurt so much.

Everything I had done counted for nothing. There was no reward at the end of this. It was heartbreak and loss, pain and suffering. We were the losers; Motor Neurone was the winner; its prize? My sister.

That night I dreamt about her. She lay in her bed her mouth so dry and sore, she was reaching for a drink but nobody gave her one. It woke me up, my own mouth felt dry, so how must hers feel? Bloody awful. She couldn't tell anyone, she couldn't write it down. I tossed and turned; her face took over my thoughts. I lay in bed silently crying in the dark so that I didn't wake Adam.

At five o'clock I went downstairs and I phoned the hospital with my concerns, but all I was told was that Diana was comfortable and that a speech therapist would see her either Monday or Tuesday, and she couldn't have anything by mouth until she had been seen. Her swallowing had to be checked first.

I'm afraid I did not agree with what she told me. So I looked up Claire's mobile number. I knew she wouldn't answer it as it was early hours Sunday morning, probably her day off. But at least I could leave a message.

As I started to speak I couldn't stop myself crying. Through my tears I told her how worried I was and how uncomfortable Diana must be not having any water. I apologised for crying and for leaving the message on her mobile but if there was anything she could do I would be so grateful.

I climbed back in bed hoping Claire would listen to my message before Monday, I knew she wouldn't be working, but I didn't know what else to do.

The very next day (Sunday) Claire phoned me. She had listened to my message then made some phone calls requesting Diana be seen ASAP, and that she should be allowed some fluid. In fact someone had the idea of ice lollies, (it was written on the board above Diana's bed when we next went in). Of course, I thought, what a good idea. It meant Diana could suck a lolly without taking in too much fluid. And she wouldn't choke.

I couldn't thank Claire enough when she phoned to tell me what she had done; it was such a weight off my mind. It was so good of her to listen to her messages especially on a Sunday and sort out my request.

The next time we visited, me, Mum, Lauren, Liam and Adam, it was so noticeable how different she looked. From when Adam and I had last seen her, her face didn't look so skeletal, it looked plumper. The fluids and the antibiotics were thankfully working; I felt such relief when I saw her. I had prepared the others for a shock but amazingly her appearance looked quite good. She sat on her bed looking so lost and lonely, the ward was full of women, and by their beds were drinks and food, it felt so unfair that my sister could have nothing by hers. The first thing Diana did was cry when she saw us; she grabbed the bag Lauren was holding. It only contained fresh clothes for her, not the precious food and drink she was so obviously looking for. As we sat there the tea trolley arrived, I asked one of the nurses if Diana could have some tea with Thick and Easy in it.

I had taken a tin in just for that purpose. I knew the hospital would have some but, I was prepared in case there wasn't any with her for when the tea trolley arrived, which there wasn't.

The nurse on duty said it was ok; it was easier to feed the tea to Diana from a teaspoon, as it was quite thick. It was so nice to see her enjoying every mouthful.

We all took turns to sit and hold her hand. I had taken in a magazine, I don't know why really, but it didn't feel right visiting and not taking her something. Lauren flicked through the pages pointing things out to her, Diana looked but only because Lauren was pointing things out to her. The magazine and its contents held no interest for her.

It was then that I noticed the list above her bed, it read custard, jelly and ice-lollies.

I remembered seeing an ice cream box at the shop near to the entrance of the hospital, so I sent Adam to buy her an ice-lolly as it would make her happy and I certainly felt good that we had something to offer her. While Adam had gone, a nurse came to her bed to check on her antibiotic bag. She then opened a bag she had with her. It contained little sticks with pink a sponge on the end, these she told us were to wipe inside and freshen Diana's mouth and remove any food particles that may be caught in her mouth; it was also to clean her tongue. Diana quite happily allowed the nurse to do this, she sat very patiently, and she seemed to enjoy the attention. And it must have made her mouth feel fresher and not so dry.

The nurse announced that she recognised Diana from school and was in the same year. Diana of course didn't show any recognition of knowing this friendly gentle person, she rubbed Diana's arm affectionately which conveyed to me how she felt, then left us.

When Adam returned with the lolly, Diana practically tore it from his hand, I had to take it back to unwrap. I then held it as she tried to suck the end, this became very messy as her mouth and tongue muscles were very weak. But did she enjoy that lolly or what! To hell with the mess!

It was great to see. As we prepared to leave we left one of the nurses holding the sticky mess. She didn't seem to mind us leaving her this time, the lovely cold delicious lolly that Diana was savouring saved us and her all the upset she usually displayed as we left her.

I knew I would be able to sleep that night, as I could see her improvement in just one day. She was recovering from her pneumonia; hopefully she could come home soon.

In all Diana stayed in hospital twelve days. Liam and Lauren managed to catch up on some much needed sleep. Although I felt guilty that Adam came in from work and without time for his dinner took us in to visit Diana, we went in every other day as it was too much for us all. Our friends Mary and Ed went in and Amanda her carer also visited so that gave us back a couple of days.

Picking her up it was obvious she was glad to be leaving. She waved to everyone in the ward and took hold of some of the nurse's hands as she went past them; they had obviously been very kind and looked after her very well.

Some hugged her, others waved, they all knew who she was.

I had collected a wheelchair from the entrance of the hospital and made her sit in it as it was quite a trek back to the car, too far for her to manage. She looked well, but I wondered how long that would last.

Arriving home I could sense how pleased she was to be back in her safe warm house. Between us we had cleaned the place top to bottom, something that rarely got done since her illness.

We had changed her bedclothes, polished furniture, washed floors, the place positively gleamed.

Diana went straight to the fridge, which made us laugh, as things were definitely back to normal, or as normal as this house could be.

Chapter 16

A few days after Diana's return Prof Coles came to see Diana. Also in the group was Jack from the disability team, the district nurse Hayley with the mad hair, Claire, Professor Cole's nurse, myself, Lauren and Amanda Diana's carer. The room was packed, it didn't bother Diana as so many people came and went, we were all used to the regular intrusions.

The first thing discussed was possible respite. Even though Diana had been in hospital for twelve days, it became full on as soon as she came home. It would give Liam and Lauren time to recharge their batteries, and sleep was a definite problem for them. The carers also became very tired as Diana's was such an unusual case. We all agreed it was definitely needed by everyone connected and involved with Diana.

Then the subject of a feeding tube was discussed. As soon as it was mentioned, Diana became agitated, she started to smack Lauren's arm and cry, she then came to me and looked at me with real fright in her eyes. 'I don't think we should discuss things in front of Diana,' I said to Prof Coles. Amanda straight away came to Diana and in her gentle voice asked if she would like to go for a ride in her car. Diana happily followed Amanda, we watched as they went to the car, but something stopped her and she turned around and came back in again, she came straight over to me. It was like from somewhere deep in her mind she knew she was being discussed and refused to leave.

'I know, Diana why don't you help Amanda make you some tea?' I suggested, with that she left the room.

'I'm not too sure about the feeding tube, you could see by Diana's reaction.' I directed this at Prof Coles.

'It would make things easier,' she replied. 'If Diana needed antibiotics again and also getting food into her.

Although I can see she has deteriorated more than I anticipated, I think at the most Diana has three months.'

I shot a look straight at Lauren, as I couldn't believe what I had just heard. Lauren burst into tears. I also couldn't hold it in either, the tears rolled down my face.

'I'm sorry, Lauren,' Prof Coles was speaking again, 'but I think you needed to know.'

If looks could kill Prof Coles would have died instantly there and then. I don't think Lauren would have batted an eyelid if she had dropped dead at her feet.

I felt angry that Prof Coles had blurted it out the way she did, especially to a sixteen-year-old who adored her mother.

Jack and Hayley looked cross but like me said nothing. There was nothing we could say.

It had come at us like a bullet, we knew it was coming but hearing it made it so final. Lauren looked shell shocked.

Diana came back into the room; she straight away noticed Lauren's puffy eyes and began to cry.

I said the first thing that came into my head. 'Lauren's got something in her eye, Diana. She's fine aren't you, Lauren?'

'Yeah, Mum, I'm ok; don't cry I'm fine.'

She is such an amazing girl. As she pulled herself together so Diana didn't pick up on the mood that was now in the room, she hugged her mum and helped her sit down on her special chair.

Prof Coles was speaking again. 'I think I will make an appointment and see how it goes.'

She was referring to the bloody feeding tube again, but this time sensibly she didn't say the word.

'And I will contact the Duchess of Kent House for respite. I'll go now, Diana. I'm sure you'll be glad to see the back of me.' Diana pointed to the front door. Yep, she wanted Prof Coles gone and so did Lauren.

Claire was next, she gave Diana a hug and left.

Hayley stood up. 'Are you ok, Lauren? I don't think it needed to come out like that,' she said.

'I'm ok,' Lauren replied.

Hayley hugged Diana and Lauren. 'I'll see you both in a few days,' she said.

She rubbed my arm as she knew I was upset. 'Thanks, Hayley, some people don't have very good bedside manners,' I said to her.

Jack got up and immediately Diana walked over to him and voluntarily hugged him. 'Oh thank you, Diana,' he said as he hugged her back.

He is such a nice guy; anyone would like Jack. He was made to do this job, it felt good that he was always at the end of the phone to sort out any problems that arose.

These people were the heroes, the ones that understood exactly what this family were going through. Even if I never see them again I will never ever forget them.

Once they had gone the atmosphere was very subdued. I could see Lauren wanting to talk about what was said but of course we couldn't say a thing until Diana was out of earshot or she fell asleep, like she sometimes did in the afternoon.

When she finally had a nap Lauren fired questions at me. I had to answer very carefully.

'I'm so sorry Prof Coles said what she did in front of you.'

I said that the life Diana was living had no quality, that I hated seeing her struggle through, day after day, suffering as she did. I said I didn't want her to suffer and that it was a blessing that Diana had Dementia because it took away the knowledge that her life would end and that she had forgotten Lauren's father as well. I told her that I believed in life after death and that she would be there watching over the two of them and be so proud of what they had both done for her. I could see that Lauren was taking all this in. She then spoke. 'I don't want my mum to suffer but it hurt so much when Prof Coles said it, I just thought I would have my mum a bit longer.'

'I know, darling,' I said, 'but the longer she lives the worse this disease will become, it is relentless. I just pray that when the time comes your mum goes peacefully in her sleep.'

As I said that my tears began to fall, as did Lauren's and Amanda's. We all stood and hugged each other. I was glad that Liam was out, he would have been inconsolable.

We carried on talking for ages. It felt good to unload how we were all feeling and the cry had relieved a lot of pent up emotions.

By the time Diana woke up we were back to near normal, she could pick on upset very easily. So we carried on as we always did, Amanda following Diana around, covering miles day after day, while I helped with washing and housework, things that Amanda had no time to do now. Even making meals for Liam and Lauren became too difficult. It was only really if Diana slept in the day that Amanda was able to make them something to eat. Diana was so wobbly now and she tended to scuff her feet as she walked and trip over, as the strength to lift her feet properly was becoming increasingly difficult for her.

We had to remove the rug in the lounge not only because it became so badly stained but she tended to trip as she tried to walk over it; it was too dangerous to leave it down any longer. Anything on the floor leading to the kitchen had to be moved in case she fell.

No longer could she wander round the house on her own; someone had to be with her at all times. It was becoming a two man job. And it was becoming impossible for the children to be out at the same time, unless mum or I were there as backup for the carer. My visits were becoming more frequent especially evenings to help shower Diana or dress her for bed, or just keep them company, a different face to sit with them and keep Lauren company and support her until Liam came in. Rita also came over regularly to keep them company.

About a week after Prof Coles' visit I received a telephone call from a nurse at the Duchess of Kent House she was a Macmillan nurse. She asked if we would like Diana to have ten days' respite towards the end of October.

I agreed straight away as already Liam and Lauren were finding it difficult again with their mother. They were worn out already even though Diana had only been back a few days, the same routine had begun again. Diana wakeful at night going from one bedroom to the next, opening and closing their doors, switching on their lights, needing help in the toilet, already it became full on again for them, night time being the worst. It wasn't fair to expect this to continue so I contacted Jack as they would need night carers very soon.

I hoped he could arrange this for when Diana returned from the Duchess of Kent.

Chapter 17

By now poor Chloe my daughter-in-law was fit to burst. John was desperate to have a boy as he said (his quote), 'All girls are whiny whinging things and are only good for one thing.' Um I wonder what he could mean? Male chauvinist! John loves football; no he's obsessed with football! Whatever you are talking about he always manages to bring footy into it. You could be talking about the weather or bicycles, he just has a knack of changing the conversation to his beloved sport. He is also quite a character, (as are his two brothers), he once took Chloe to the hospital because she was experiencing some pain and believed it was the start of labour, because they had such a long wait and things weren't happening he decided to tie Chloe's legs together and then to the bed because he was bored. Where he got the string I have no idea! He then climbed on the bed next to her because he felt tired, much to the nurses' disgust when they came to check on her. As it happened it was a false alarm, much to John's disgust.

They had a few more false alarms. Every time I gave Chloe a hug and wished her well, back they would come after being told it won't be long and be patient. If Chloe got any bigger she would explode like a balloon that had been blown too high and would burst any minute. Her poor tummy was quite large.

Finally on 22nd October 2010 Rianne June Diana was born. Unusual choice for middle names I know, Diana as a tribute to my sister and June after John's late Grandma. Rianne weighed a whopping 10lb 7ozs. I could not believe her weight as John is quite a small chap and so is Chloe, so the rumours jokingly flew round that she couldn't possibly be John's and must be the football team's goalkeeper's baby, him being well over six-foot. By the size Chloe got to I am convinced and so was Chloe that her dates were wrong. Once I saw Rianne she didn't look the weight they said although the scales didn't lie. She was very swollen; once the swelling went down I know I am biased but what a beautiful baby she has turned out to be. Lovely big blue eyes and a dimple one side of her cheek and a little character just as her father had been. John taught her at a very young age to cough when Chloe went outside for a cigarette. It is very funny when you say to her, 'Have you got a bad cough, Rianne?' and as ordered she gives a false cough just as her daft Dad taught her. John's way of saying to Chloe, 'Give up the fags.'

She mimics very well and talks with her eyes; the expressions are funny, the looks she gives are hilarious.

I know for a fact that once she begins to talk properly she will be exactly as her father was; question after question. 'What, why, how, where, when, who, but, why.' It didn't matter what answer I gave John it was never the right one; his mind whirred continuously with question after question. Seeing how bright Rianne is she will be the same as her father.

He will have a taste of how he was as a young boy. Good luck, John!

Chapter 18

We received an appointment for Diana to attend the Royal Berks Hospital. This I was dreading because I knew Diana would not entertain a feeding tube and it would be a wasted, stressful journey for her.

But we went as requested and as soon as she saw the hospital she began to cry. It took a lot of persuading to get her out of the car.

When finally in the waiting room she kept pulling at Lauren's hand to indicate she wanted to leave. The waiting room luckily was empty, so we didn't have to wait too long.

The nurse took us into a room where she started to explain about the feeding tube to Diana.

You're wasting your time, I thought. She won't know what the hell you are talking about.

She was holding the tube to show Diana. Diana smacked the nurse's arm away, and began to shake her head and cry, making groaning noises. These were all she could do now; she turned away from the nurse and shuffled out the way we came in.

Lauren followed to steady her, while I talked to the nurse.

'If Diana didn't have Dementia then I'm sure she would agree to the feeding tube,' I said to the nurse, 'but if we went ahead it would be forced upon her. I don't think I can make that decision for her, you saw her reaction when you showed her the tube, she was frightened because she doesn't understand.'

'I don't think this is a good idea,' she agreed with me. 'Once the tube is fitted Diana may try and pull it out, and that is very dangerous,' the nurse stated.

There was no may about it; I knew she would pull it out.

The nurse suggested we went away and thought about it as she needed to speak to the doctor who performed the procedure.

I agreed to ring her in a few days, to find out the doctor's opinion and give our answer. I knew that already but I said I would phone her.

At home we discussed it between ourselves when Diana was sleeping; Mum had come round to help out as usual, with housework etc. I must say we worked bloody hard, to keep everything up together, as the washing was endless. Mum would bring her shopping trolley with her and load it with piles of dirty washing to take back with her, as some days we couldn't keep up with the amount of washing that appeared every day. We changed bedclothes and cleaned so the house stayed reasonably smart for the never-ending hoards of visitors. Diana would want it like that, she had always been very house proud.

We waited for Diana to sleep then talked about the bloody feeding tube.

I spoke first. 'It will be against her will and she won't understand why we are putting her through it.'

My mum nodded in agreement. 'I think it would be too distressing for her,' Mum said.

'I don't want my mum frightened,' Lauren said, 'and I wouldn't know what to do if Mum tried to pull it out.'

It was usually left to me to make the final decision, but I still needed everyone's opinions as to whether I was making the right one.

It was such a huge task to make these kinds of decisions. Diana was a very sick girl, what if I made the wrong choice?

But realistically I knew it was the only choice I could make, Diana without Dementia would have agreed without any question, but she did have it.

We couldn't take the risk that she may pull it out. She would be hospitalised again and going through yet more stress, and a possible serious operation. I just didn't know.

So when Monday came I rang the nurse and told her our decision. She told me that the doctor had already said it was too big a risk to put her through. That made me feel so much better as I was preparing myself for a battle with them as to why she shouldn't have one fitted.

So the feeding tube was forgotten about and never mentioned again. We couldn't spend our days going through what ifs etc., we had so little time left with her, we couldn't dwell over what might have been.

By the end of October everyone was exhausted and snappy with each other. We all needed the respite, to once again recharge our depleted batteries. It was someone else's turn to look after Diana so we could be the visitors and spend quality time with her, without all the hard work that went with her illness.

It was agreed that Amanda and Liam would take Diana to the Duchess of Kent. I had helped the night before to pack Diana's things and medication; she didn't seem to notice as we brought these items down stairs.

A nurse from the Duchess of Kent had phoned me and requested we bring the sucker machine with us.

In the morning Diana got in Amanda's car quite happily as to Diana Amanda and her car meant nice trips out. Our car usually meant hospital trips, which caused Diana so much distress and agitation.

I felt mean that we were tricking Diana and that it was left to Amanda, but she was so kind and loving to Diana, her patience was remarkable. Diana never hit Liam like she sometimes did Lauren, so he went along as Amanda's support.

It was almost like Diana somewhere remembered Liam had learning difficulties and it was Lauren she sometimes had her battles with. It was usually about Lauren moaning how her hair wasn't right or her shoes didn't feel right. Lauren herself will remember the days I got phone calls from Diana saying Lauren was upset about something or other and could she come over until Lauren's outburst had calmed down. But they always made up and were friends again until the next problem arose. It was also because they were so close and so alike that they did have these mother-daughter disagreements. Liam just went with the flow, in his own quiet way.

Once they reached the duchess of Kent they both found it hard leaving her with the nurses as she became upset when it was time for them to leave.

From her spell in hospital to now October, Diana's appearance had changed again. Her neck muscles had become weaker, this made her head sit to the right, against her right shoulder. Just to lift it was a terrible struggle for her. Sat down she could hold it back against the chair and look straight ahead, but as soon as she stood up to walk about her head lolled sideways. The changes in her were now happening rapidly. My heart ached for her but I had to keep upbeat, and hide the anger and upset I felt to myself. Inside I wanted to scream and hit out. 'WHY ARE YOU DOING THIS TO MY SISTER YOU FUCKING BASTARD DISEASE?'

But there was no one to yell at. God wasn't hearing me, there was no one to bargain or plead with.

Day by day we were losing her and it hurt like hell.

One of the nurses at the Duchess of Kent had requested that we didn't visit Diana the first night, 'So she can settle in,' we were told.

Adam and I had visited the Duchess of Kent a few weeks prior to her stay. It wasn't like a hospital but a warm and cosy home. There were clean wooden floorboards along the corridors and paintings on the walls, beautiful drapes at the windows adding to the cosiness, a room for families to gather when they visited their loved ones. I noticed a piano and comfortable chairs and settees to sit on; plants here and there completed the look. Outside, the gardens looked lovingly tended with bird tables, and seats to relax on. It felt so homely, great care had been taken to make the right atmosphere so patients could relax in their rooms and the visitors' lounge. It wasn't like a hospital, it was only the fact that the nurses wore uniforms that made you realise it was a medical place. The rooms were spacious with wardrobes and an en-suite toilet; each room had a telly and a comfortable leather chair for patients to sit on. The bed could be moved up and down front and back to suit the patient's needs, the bed covers were brightly coloured and brightened the room. Diana could no longer lie down so the bed could be raised at the head and also the middle so that the whole body could be made comfortable.

I must admit the place impressed me; I had no worries at her staying there.

It was with great apprehension the very next night that we made our way through heavy traffic. Although it wasn't too far away it was always going to be busy when we left our homes to visit Diana. By the time Adam got home to pick us up, the traffic was pretty bumper to bumper for him to then have to turn round and go back out in to it.

I felt guilty as he had no time to eat, and was always tired after a long day on the road calling on various customers in many counties. He never once complained but made space for Liam and Lauren in our car, we then collected them and set off on our journey.

As soon as Diana saw us she began to cry, she immediately took Lauren by the arm and shuffled from her room along the corridor towards the front door, there she tried to unlock it.

She shook the door with her good arm then pointed at it. Diana was indicating she wanted to go home, Lauren led her back along the corridor, talking to her to try and distract her from the front door. There was a little sitting area by the nurses' reception, it had two comfortable leather settees a telly and a table with various items that could be bought by patients and visitors. There was also a box to put money in for the goods purchased, it was all done on trust. It was easy then to distract Diana from the front door, as we took her to look at all the gifts that were on sale. Picking them up one by one then replacing them very carefully, this was a very good distraction. There were greetings cards and small cuddly bears, writing pads, and pens, pencils, wallets, purses and lucky charms.

It became a ritual with Diana that we brought her something from the gift table each time we visited. She still made her way to the front door, quite a few times during the time we were there, but we just turned her round chatting to her the whole time taking her mind from the pesky door, making our way back to the little table of treasures then on to her room.

One thing I had discussed with the nurses were her bowels; of course! I needed to know they were continuing with her medicine and that she wasn't uncomfortable. I was assured that Diana had in fact emptied them that day and I wasn't to worry. Not worry, that was a laugh, it was all I did and all I had done for the last two years. My worry lines had become grooves were getting deeper by the day!

I don't think I have relaxed properly since October 2007. Even away on holiday my mind went over everything that I left behind, it was difficult to forget even so far away. It was only sleep that took away the constant thoughts and worries.

Lauren also had a constant headache, it I knew to be worry and stress. Headache tablets didn't help her, it was the situation we were living in. We didn't want it, we couldn't get rid of it, it couldn't be forgotten about, it was with us and there it stayed day after day and for Liam and Lauren night after night, relentlessly wearing us down. No drugs would heal it. Prof Coles was an expert in its field but there was no treatment and no cure. Not much to be an expert in really! I was learning so much about this disease, its unfairness and destruction. The possibility of only having between two and five years before death, drugs that help one problem cause a whole load more. It also takes a long time before Motor Neurone is diagnosed as other possibilities are eliminated, although in Diana's case I understood why it took so long to diagnose considering what had happened to her since Sean had left. We were all sure it was the effect of him leaving.

I know all the drugs off by heart, what they did or in some cases didn't do; in fact they really did sod all. They may have helped initially a tiny bit, but further along the illness took a vice-like grip of her body. With each medicine came a side effect. One of these medicines was Atropine, which is in fact an eye drop treatment; they found it could help with the incessant dribbling. But of course as with most of her medications it caused other problems. The drops were placed on the tongue but it caused her saliva to congeal into large green phlegm balls at the back of her throat. Her swallowing was so bad now that these could cause choking as she had no way of coughing them up herself. They caused Diana to struggle to breathe and she could not clear her throat as you or I. There was no way she could swallow the big green sticky gunge balls. This was the most frightening thing Diana had to experience.

We decided to stop the Atropine ourselves as one of Diana's choking fits was so bad and frightened us all. She had started to cough as she regularly did due to the never ending mucous; it was obvious that this was more serious than usual. I grabbed the yanker and pushed it as far into Diana's throat as I could which wasn't easy as she struggled gasping for breath. Lauren was holding her hands to stop her smacking my hands away and Katherine was trying to hold her head still.

I could see this large green blob, it was blocking her airway. As I touched the back of her throat with the tube it made Diana retch and as she did I managed to suck it all away. The disgusting congealed blob made its way along the tube and into the container.

Diana was shaking and crying. It was so unfair that she should have to go through episodes like these. Lauren was upset and shaking and I just plonked down on the chair in utter relief shaking like jelly. That was the last time we used Atropine, its side effect was too dangerous.

Letting the saliva flow free didn't seem so bad now. It was a real pain for Diana for her clothes, her carpets and her constantly wet chest but nothing compared to that awful incident.

Diana's stay at the Duchess of Kent was good for everyone. The nurses were wonderful with her, one of the nurses Diana really took a shine to she followed her around each day as she came on duty. They did her hair into a French plait so that it stayed clean and wasn't continually matted with food as it was at home. (She wouldn't let us tie her hair back at home.) They changed her constantly so that when we went in she looked clean and fresh. She let them shower her as their caring and gentle ways made Diana like and trust them. It was so nice for us to just sit with her without tending to all the horrors Motor Neurone brought with it. We watched telly with her, walked around the corridors with her and I held her hand and stroked it; something she liked. She still cried when she first saw us but we made a big fuss of her every time we arrived, chatting away to her about everyday things but avoiding mentioning home as every visit gave her hope we had come to fetch her home. It felt good to spend quality time with her and not spend every waking moment worrying about her.

Because they were so very good with Diana, I for once actually felt myself relax; she was in a good place with lovely caring people. There were no panic calls to her doctor as everything she needed the Duchess of Kent could supply. Liam and Lauren were able to sleep again, and see their friends when they wanted and come and go as they pleased.

Although hard, the visits were enjoyable, Diana still walked us backwards and forwards to the locked front door trying the handle each time, and she still cried over the slightest thing and hated it when we left, but we knew she was being looked after in a way that we had not been able to. That made leaving her easier, they could deal with any choking fits, they were trained and they had the right equipment to deal with problems that may arise during her stay. Her room was comfortable and the staff were wonderful.

In all Diana stayed fourteen days. She actually looked quite well even though her body was skin and bone. It suited her with her hair tied back in a neat plait, but as soon as she was home she wouldn't have it any way but down. This caused more problems as her hair became tangled due to food bits and the lack of washing and brushing. It was only Amanda that she allowed to brush it and very carefully try to detangle it. Trying to wash it made her hit out and cry. I think she found it distressing, again part of the mysteries of Dementia. She became cross if Lauren made it wet in the shower, so her hair was left alone apart from the occasional brushing. It didn't really matter now; just keeping her happy and comfortable, they were our main concerns.

Because of Diana's lack of fluids and my fear she could be hospitalised again, I requested if possible that she be rehydrated at home. I needed her and the children to have their last Christmas together, with her as well and as happy as possible.

It is so painful writing this bit, as it was to be her last Christmas, her last time to be there for the games I arranged. To win the prizes I brought especially for each game. The last Christmas dinner together, never to see her face again, or hear her giggle when she got the answers wrong, as she often did. Never to tease her again because she did get them wrong or tell her off for cheating. Next Christmas will have a huge personality missing and it will be so sad that she has gone with no other sister or brother to fill that gap, to share the upset and hurt, to understand how I was feeling about losing a loved one.

Chapter 19

While Diana had been in respite Liam and Lauren had been busy. On their own they decorated the house with Christmas decorations, the place looked amazing. They had covered the tree in lights and they had done it all exactly as Diana used to. Everything had its place, just as she had done in previous years. Tinsel draped over the pictures in the lounge and dining room, a golden garland along the mantelpiece with red candles either end, the nativity next to the telly as it always was, the nodding reindeer lit up in the front garden. Everything as Diana would have arranged it. The icicle lights hanging from the garage porch twinkling in the dark. The house looked amazing inside and out.

All done by my amazing niece and nephew, God bless them both.

Diana's eyes said it all as she looked around when she first entered her beautifully decorated home; she walked from room to room and decoration to decoration touching them almost as if she were checking them over. She stood staring at the tree almost mesmerized, touching the sparkling baubles, letting her fingers run along the soft shining tinsel. How much did she remember? Did she remember Christmas? Did she even know it was December? I didn't think so but she seemed to like what she saw. It brightened the place and gave it warmth; her illness had made it cold for so long. How could anyone have a problem at such a special time of year? And yet here we all were waiting to celebrate what was Diana's most favourite time of the year, and sadly her last.

How angry she would have been if she had known how ill she was and that it was robbing her of so many wonderful times ahead.

My request was granted, Diana would be rehydrated at home; it made it less stressful for Diana and too much for her to go into hospital again. The nurses had to come in every other day anyway to give Diana her suppositories, so there were plenty of medical staff coming and going if there should be any problems.

I had been rushing around the weeks leading up to Christmas. I had my own Christmas shopping to do, then Mum's as she wasn't up to shopping for presents and then there were the presents from Diana to her children. Three lots of shopping and two adults is a lot of shopping and not enough adults, but it couldn't be helped. I feel sure I must have been a donkey in a previous life as we were loaded down like one. Three lists and one pen to mark off each pressie purchased, also three separate purses so I didn't mix the money up.

All this done at Basingstoke's indoor shopping centre Festival Place; the kind of place I didn't really like, hot, humid too many people! Done on two separate Saturdays, which I think is pretty good going. I absolutely loathe shopping, any kind, we even managed to stop and eat lunch in between. I hate queuing up, I hate waiting and I hate shoppers that dither and window shop and here I was doing three loads and waiting in queues, and dithering and window shopping. At least I had got my niece and nephew to write down what they wanted, as I had no idea what a sixteen-year-old girl was into and I couldn't risk choosing her clothing. Liam was a bit easier as having boys myself it was roughly the same for him: jeans, t-shirts, CDs, DVDs, lots of sweets, and smellies and of course Christmas wouldn't be Christmas without a six pack of socks, preferably with daft sayings on or days of the week; the usual thing. A couple of pairs of Ben Sherman boxers and Liam was done.

Lauren wrote down names and makes and requested something I had never heard of, jeggings! A cross between leggings and jeans I was told, actually a very good idea now I've seen some. She also pointed out the type of jeans she wore and where to get them from, that was a help as there are now so many styles. Skinny! Super skinny! Straight leg, flair, bootleg, hipsters! God my brain hurts!! My Mum didn't actually have a list she just told me to choose what I thought everyone would like. Even harder!

I stuck to a few well known stores like New look and Next for clothes, H.M.V. for CDs and DVDs, so I didn't have to traipse around looking for the best deals.

Super drug for smellies and Sports World for reasonably priced trackies etc. I wasn't going to go from shop to shop to compare prices, not this time anyway. Time was precious and I was always aware that any moment Adam's phone may ring with a problem concerning Diana so the quicker the shopping was done the better.

I then had the task of wrapping up my ones and then the ones from Diana. It would take forever, so I did a few every day, as it's another little job I detest. Pressie wrapping; all that effort to then be ripped apart in five seconds.

Why I wasn't falling asleep on my feet I don't know, as I was sleeping so badly at night. It must have been adrenaline that kept me going, funny really because people always say how tired Adam looks but never me and yet I felt exhausted. I told this to my friend and she agreed I looked the picture of health and yes Adam's bags under his eyes were bigger than Sainsbury's. Not that I minded, it would just have been nice for someone to say, 'Oh dear, Jan you do look tired. I'll do that, you go and put your feet up for an hour,' but no, I looked un-tired and obviously fit to go not drop! Don't get me wrong, Liam, Lauren and Mum were all exhausted, it was go all the time, more so for the two kids.

Of course once all the pressies were bought, it was then the food that had to be thought about. As we were the only ones free and with a car it again became mine and Adam's task to get in all that was needed for Christmas.

Reading it back now I sound sarcastic. I know my sister would never have burdened me with all this or my mum. It wasn't their fault and I would do it every day if it gave me back my sister and made my mum well.

The nurses were coming in three days before Christmas to put Diana on her rehydration thingamabob. The trouble with doing this at home (I found out from the nurse that came) was the drip line was very thin so Diana was only getting a few mils a minute. The fluid in the bag hanging on an old coat hanger, stuck over a picture above Diana's chair was only going to drain slightly and very slowly. Not much fluid was going into Diana. I suppose some was better than none.

Another problem was when Diana got up someone had to grab the coat hanger and follow her, bag and all, (before she ripped the lot off the wall). She did of course constantly get up and go on her walkabout followed by whoever managed to grab the coat hanger first. Usually the nearest to her chair at the time.

This all seemed a bit like a Carry On film to me. I know this was being done at my request but was it really worth the effort? But it was too late to change now. I just hoped more fluid would go in than the expected dose. And Diana getting up and down from her chair every few minutes was even harder work for the carers, and when they went at eight p.m. I then joined Liam and Lauren until ten p.m. to help as it was so exhausting. Where Diana's energy came from I really didn't have a clue, but no sooner had you sat her down then up she would get again. When the nurse came to remove the drip it was a relief.

As stated the fluid hardly moved (what a waste of time but done with good intention). We had to give Diana ice pops to suck on, not only for her dry mouth but also to try and occupy her and encourage her to sit for a while, just to give us all a rest from jumping up and grabbing the coat hanger before she pulled it and the picture down.

I am amazed that with so little in her body she had the strength to walk around as much as she did, her determination was astounding and completely knackering for us! Why the pounds didn't drop off me I shall never fathom, I'm obviously not meant to be the beanpole I used to be.

The nurse arrived the next day at about ten a.m. and said another nurse would be back at ten p.m. to remove it. And so the cycle continued.

Christmas Eve was the worst day of all; the nurse had arrived as usual and attached Diana to the drip, I had gone with Mum's food list and a list for Liam and Lauren, to buy Christmas food from Sainsbury's. (I don't remember why I had left it so late to food shop as I am usually done the day before Christmas Eve.) I had decided to go back and do mine afterwards as we had so much to buy. Adam and I hoped to have lunch and then leisurely take a bit of time to do my shopping, knowing that the carer was helping the kids.

I delivered my mother's shopping, then as we turned into Diana's road with her shopping, we saw Lauren coming towards us, she came over to our car.

'Is everything ok at home?'

'Yeah,' Lauren replied, 'Liam's there with Mum. I'm going to see my friend.'

'Where's the carer?' I asked.

'She had to go because there was nobody to pick up her son from school.'

'But Liam can't stay on his own with your mum it's a two person job with the drip in,' I barked at her. 'And I've still got to go and do my shopping. Is anyone else coming?'

By now Lauren was looking very tearful. I didn't mean to snap at her but a replacement carer should have been sent. Liam could not manage his mother and a drip and tend to her frequent toilet visits on his own. He was a lad, it wasn't fair for a boy to do those, and as I stated this was now a two man job. He was marvellous with everything but I couldn't be in two places at once. I hadn't done my own shop yet, I felt panic rise as the shops would close early today.

'God what a mess,' I said out loud.

'I'll come back,' Lauren said reluctantly.

'No, love, that's not the point. These people are being paid to look after your mum, it's not good enough. You deserve a bit of freedom to see your friends.'

I felt so angry, if I didn't get back to the shops Christmas day would consist of a turkey and little else.

Poor Liam was holding on to his mother's drip as she walked backwards and forwards from room to room. He told me that he had been asked by the carer if she could go home because there was no one to collect her son from school. What could the poor lad say? It should never have been left to him to make that decision. (She should have notified her boss and asked for a replacement, that's if one could have been found at such short notice.) I had no choice but to phone Jack. Luckily he was still at work, I told him what had happened. He was very cross and apologetic, as I explained I still had food shopping to do for myself, and that Lauren once again had to come back and cancel her friends and that it was too dangerous for Liam to cope with his mother's needs. 'I will try and get someone to you,' he told me.

'Look, Jack, I don't mind coming back later but I must get my shopping done.'

As soon as I put the phone down I burst into tears, this of course made Diana cry and Lauren and Liam looked very upset. Liam hugged me. 'I'm sorry, Aunty Jan,' he said.

'It's not your fault, Liam but some days I don't know which way to turn.'

I pulled myself together as I didn't want to upset them anymore than I had already done, and poor Diana didn't know why I was crying. 'Lauren can you just wait ten minutes until the replacement carer comes? Then you go out as planned and meet your friends, I will come back for the evening to help out until the nurses come to remove your mum's drip.'

Diana stopped crying because I did, she just wasn't aware of all that was going on. Poor girl.

So I did my shopping at a rush because the replacement carer could only stay until four o'clock. And instead of preparing my vegetables Christmas Eve and laying the table, and putting out the crackers and serviettes in the glasses and place names, I spent my evening taking turns with Lauren who returned at seven p.m. (because Liam was going out), jumping up and down grabbing Diana's drip and following her as usual from room to room or feeding her ice-cream or yogurts in between toilet visits.

Between us we made light of it. What else could we do? Our lives were so extreme now; things could not and would not be normal while Diana needed so much from us.

Adam now had the job of peeling my veg and laying the table, thank goodness he is such an easy going bloke, he has made my life so much easier, these last three years. He has been my rock; without his support I would never have coped with what has been happening to our family.

Usually on Christmas Eve in my home we would watch any good Christmassy programmes that were on, but Diana was now no longer interested in telly, so Lauren and I spent a lot of the evening talking and walking from room to room, (even upstairs sometimes), taking turns to carry the coat hanger.

We gave Diana her medicines at the usual time and sort of watched a bit of telly, but we were so completely knackered by the time the nurses arrived at ten, we then had to get Diana into the shower and dress her for bed. Because of her bad arm we had to go so carefully when dressing her, this always took a little while, so when I wasn't there it must have taken poor Lauren ages. Diana didn't want to go to bed while I was there, so Lauren said she would get ready for bed and then lay next to her mother so that Diana would hopefully fall asleep.

I felt bad leaving her but it was getting on for eleven p.m. and I felt shattered, and Adam was waiting for my phone call to pick me up. He got very tired these days since his heart attack so I had to consider him as well. I hoped Liam wouldn't be late as it was usually Lauren that drew the short straw. He promised her he wouldn't be late in, and I hoped he would keep to his word.

I didn't go straight to bed when I got in as the carrots Adam had prepared looked like door stops and were more for burly rugby players and not an ordinary family sitting down to a turkey dinner. I also had to finish off my place names as I always had silly names at dinner. Last year I had Adolf Hitler, Peggy Mitchell, the queen, Jessica Simpson, Del Boy, Rudolph Hess, and Cher. I think it made it more fun and the visitors seemed to enjoy it. (Truth be known I find it funny regardless of what my guests think) I also if I have time make my own crackers out of loo roll holders and write my own jokes. I love Christmas and want it to be fun for everyone. This year was going to be sad but I wanted Liam and Lauren to enjoy the day.

We had decided that my dad should come to my house along with John, Chloe; baby Rianne, James, Mark, Adam and myself. Liam, Lauren, my mum and Diana should stay at Diana's house as the problem was the food and eating it without upsetting her. Diana's would have to be pureed this I knew she would not like, and because of Diana's Dementia she wouldn't understand why she couldn't have a proper Christmas dinner like everyone else.

Mum told us later that it did prove to be a problem as Diana kept trying to grab the food from the plates as my mother tried to dish up, she wouldn't be distracted by Lauren as I'm sure the smells alone were driving her mad.

Liam and Lauren had their dinner while Mum fed Diana her pureed one. In fact the two children gobbled theirs down on a tray in the lounge so as not to distress Diana, and Mum ate hers alone while Lauren fed Diana a yogurt in front of the telly. It wasn't much fun at our house either as we ate, all of us subdued, all of us aware how sad this Christmas was. Usually my dad would crack a few jokes and John would chatter away but not this year. In the past our Christmases were always full of noise, fun and teasing, jokes and loud chatting, everyone trying to be heard, but sadly not this time, we ate our dinner in silence. I was glad when it was over, and relieved to be clearing the table and washing the dishes with Adam's help.

The phone rang. It was Mum; she was concerned because Diana now had diarrhoea, and she was crying and very upset. I was surprised as she had been a bit constipated the day before. I was now worried she was having too much of her laxative medicine. The only choice I had was to phone the doctors. I don't know why but I just knew that Christmas Day something would happen. I so wanted to play the games as we always had because I wanted Diana to be included. Knowing this was her last Christmas it was so very important to me and especially to Liam and Lauren and the rest of our family.

One by one we went over to Diana's; she was still crying.

Mum told me she was refusing to sit down and getting very agitated about it. We tried to make her comfortable but she became more and more distressed and would not sit. I asked her if she was sore she just looked at me and nodded her head, but she always nodded her head when asked a question so I wasn't sure what to do. She tried to sit next to me but immediately lifted her bottom up and she squeezed my arm, looking at me with her big green scared eyes.

'Could she be sore? Should I apply some cream?' I asked our mother. I had to do something.

I took her upstairs where I put on a rubber glove and carefully applied some Sudacream; her back was so bony I could feel the bottom of her spine. It made me shudder with shock. The cream didn't seem to help as she still refused to sit down, she kept looking at me. I could see by her distressed expression she was trying to tell me something.

'What about a shower?' I said.

'But the doctor is due,' my mum replied.

'Oh sod the doctor; I can't think what else we can do. The doctor could be ages.'

How glad am I that I insisted she had a shower. We got her undressed, me, mum and Lauren. We helped her into the shower; I made sure the temperature felt right before I helped her under the spray. I then directed the spray onto her sore backside thinking it would soothe her, as I was spraying her she reached round with her good arm and began pulling at her bottom, and as she did small round and extremely hard lumps started falling from her back passage and plopping on the bath floor. Now I knew what it was: she couldn't sit because her constipation was so bad and her bowel so full it hurt her to sit. She must have been terribly uncomfortable. I can't tell you how relieved we were. Lauren went to her bedroom gagging. We laughed at Lauren; anything like this she couldn't cope with but it really didn't matter. Diana's problem was sorted, I picked up the offending lumps with my rubber glove and tissue and threw them happily into the loo, we then gave her a relaxing shower. We carefully helped her out and as I wrapped the towel around her frail thin body she looked more like an eighty-year-old woman than a youthful forty-eight year-old. She took my arm with her good hand and squeezed it. As I looked up at her I could see the thanks as her eyes looked into mine, something she hadn't done for ages. She was speaking to me with her eyes, my sister for the first time in ages had communicated with me, I had helped her and she said thank you. My eyes welled with tears.

'You're welcome, Diana,' I said. 'Now come on, let's go start the games before that doctor arrives.'

Maybe I should have left the above out of my story as it is very explicit, but it is part of Diana's story and how much she had to go through, and how we dealt with it to keep her as comfortable as we could.

The doctor did take ages to arrive and apologised for being so long but that it had been a hectic Christmas Day. When I told him the story he congratulated me for using my common sense, and that the diarrhoea we thought she had at first often happens when people become constipated. It is only liquid that breaks through giving the appearance of an upset tummy, which is why we assumed wrong.

He examined Diana anyway and said her back passage felt pretty clear. I liked him as he was so friendly. He didn't try to hurry away, but chatted to me and Diana for quite a while, asking many questions about Diana's condition and were we receiving enough help with care etc. He ended the conversation by saying not to hesitate to phone again if he was needed. He was such a lovely gentle man my sister liked right away and didn't mind him examining her.

All I know is I felt relieved that she was ok and another problem sorted, funny thing is quite a few times when I called in the following days Diana would pull my arm and lead me to the bathroom for a shower whatever the time, although she wasn't constipated now because the suppositories had been doing their stuff. She still connected me with the shower and the relief she must have felt. It was difficult persuading her that she didn't need a shower until bedtime and I would come back later if she wanted. Other times I gave in and showered her; I think the warm water warmed her thin body as now it was impossible to bath her. She would need special equipment and people who knew what they were doing.

If it made her feel happy then we did it. I won't lie some days we were at each other's throats through sheer frustration and exhaustion, and the guilt I felt at leaving Liam and Lauren on their own when there were no night time carers was immense.

Adam and I spent Boxing Day with them. We didn't eat anything, Lauren and Liam picked on nibbles in the kitchen but I had no appetite for food. It didn't feel right when Diana could eat so little. I sent Adam home to get himself something and then take the dogs out, while I helped with Diana and her constant travelling backwards and forwards. For someone so frail and mal-nourished, she had a strong heart and even stronger determination.

Before her illness she had always been strong willed and determined, she had run the home and made most of the decisions. The children must have missed the order and routine that she gave them. Also the love and security she showed them. Their lives had taken a complete turn around. A family of four one day, foundlings the next. This Diana was not the mother they knew or wanted, they still loved her very much but it was the old Diana we all craved to see and hear again; the kind, loving, and generous one that loved a laugh. Our Diana had left us the day she found out about the affair. It has been difficult to remember her, while we look after this Diana. It is hard to lose someone when they die but it is even harder to lose them while they are still alive. We try to be the same people for her sake but inside the hurt is unbearable.

Her looks had changed. Motor Neurone had aged her well beyond her years; she looked more like an eighty-year-old than a youthful forty-eight. Curse the disease, I loathed it.

Chapter 20

We made it through Christmas. It was a relief when the carers returned to take a bit of pressure away from the children, but night times even with carers were still too tiring for them. Diana was determined at all costs to get into one of their bedrooms. It would have meant the carers forcibly stopping Diana from entering their rooms which they were not allowed to do, and even with locks on the doors Diana would make wailing noises and try to open them up, continuously rattling the doors. Lauren found it too distressing to hear her mother so on nights like these she relented and let her mother in. The two of them would then squash in a tiny single bed, although it wasn't long before Diana went walk about again. By now Lauren was looking exhausted, her eyes looked constantly puffy and she was getting cold after cold because she was so run down from lack of sleep. Their eating was suffering as well, as they could only manage food when their mother slept, which could be anytime of the day. Luckily the school were aware how bad things were at home. I had rung and told Lauren's head of house that her attending school at the moment was impossible for her, as the lack of sleep was making her ill. The district nurse Hayley had commented how tired she was looking. Later that day she rang me at home.

'Don't get upset, Jan,' she started off, 'but have you considered putting Diana in a care home? Her needs are so much greater now and Lauren poor mite looks exhausted.'

'I know, Hayley. Oh, God, I can't make that decision on my own. I must ask them and Mum for their opinion. They must have a say in what happens to her.'

Talking about such a drastic but much needed step upset me greatly; everyone had done such a good job at looking after Diana I felt it would be letting her down, but I knew the children couldn't cope anymore. They were the ones taking the brunt of everything going on at home. It was going to be difficult to even broach the subject; even thinking about it brought a lump to my throat. It was also saying this was the final part of the journey. Once Diana left the family home she would never come back. Did we really want Diana to die at home? Was a care home the way forward? I knew I couldn't cope with seeing her pass away at home. I didn't want any more suffering for her and what would the end be like? I couldn't bear to think about it. I knew it would be dreadful for Liam and Lauren to see their mother pass away possibly fighting for breath. I couldn't even contemplate how awful it might be when the day did finally arrive.

One thing that had been set in place was if Diana had a heart attack did we want her to be revived and if she stopped breathing should the hospital intervene or let her go peacefully? Lauren, Mum and myself had no doubts. We wanted no suffering; she was going through enough. We made our decision, I then had to sign a letter prepared by her doctor that there was to be no intervention. The doctor then requested I buy a secure locking box, in which would be placed drugs so that in the event of the above happening these would ensure Diana did not suffer. I then had to put it in a safe place. I chose the top of one of Diana's kitchen cupboards. It could be seen but it was out of reach if any one became curious.

Even as I write this now I still can't believe it is my sister I am writing about. I haven't really had time to sit and think how much has happened and question why the hell had it happened. She was such a big part of our lives, a missing piece of our family's jigsaw that will never be replaced. I have to keep busy so I don't dwell too much as the anger and hurt starts to rise. It doesn't do any good; it won't bring her back to us. It's like a bad dream and one day I will wake up and everything will be as it was. But then I wake up and it's a nightmare and real and it is happening. Writing this is letting out my frustration, and sadness. It is her story and her children's. It's night time I hate. I can't sleep so I watch telly or read because if I don't, I think about her all the time. Could I have done more? Made her life a little sweeter? I remember sitting next to her, thinking I want this to end now. I hated seeing her so ill and I wanted her to go peacefully and soon, no more suffering. I know I didn't have the right to wish things to end, but we had all had enough. She had had enough. Human beings can be strong but we had nothing left, we were all running on empty, and Diana needed to be at rest. It wasn't our Diana anymore, the Motor Neurone and Dementia had made sure of that, it took her a little each day. I felt cross for thinking like that but an animal would not be allowed to suffer. This country needs to change its law when it comes to human suffering. It's not murder to release someone from a living hell, it would be a humane act just as with an animal. If this is a free country then where is freedom of choice. I don't know what I believed before Diana became ill but I know what I believe now!

How would the pro life people feel if one of their family were struck down with a similar or same illness? I think of her suffering, her loss of dignity, her lack of quality of life, her pain. I know because of her Dementia none of us could have made the decision to end her life for her (if a law was passed) but what of others aware of all that is going on, and praying the end will come soon without suffering and without pain. But not having that choice when it becomes unbearable, to me it is cruel.

I decided to talk to Jack about Hayley's conversation concerning Diana, her needs and those of the children. He agreed that we should meet but he needed to contact another department to have Diana assessed, because the funding would come from West Berkshire Health Care, at the moment it was half and half. Diana had little money and being on benefits including Disability Living Allowance, the care she needed could not be paid for by her meagre income. Then there was the problem of Diana's two illnesses. What care home could cater for Motor Neurone and Dementia? This it proved was going to be harder than I thought.

At the meeting were Jack, Ali from West Berks Primary Trust, a Macmillan nurse called Ellen, Hayley and Sue the district nurses and Diana's doctor, also Lauren, Liam, myself and Amanda. It was quite sombre as we sat and talked. Diana didn't take much notice she was so used to hordes of people cramming into her lounge. As she recognised a face she would lift her weak arm and wave to that person; it was really sweet. She especially liked Jack, and I couldn't think of anyone that wouldn't like him. As soon as I had first met him it was obvious he loved his job, he was good at it, and he cared about people and in that type of job you had to like people – you had to care!. He never minded me bombarding him with phone calls and anything I requested or problems that arose, as they did all the time, he did his utmost to sort it out.

Ali said she didn't think there would be a problem for the funding but it was agreed that Diana would need one to one care. This also had to be funded because she was so active and spent a lot of time on her feet scuffling around. She couldn't be allowed to wander on her own. It wasn't safe and very dangerous if she fell.

As I sat there listening I looked at Liam and Lauren's sad faces. It was awful for them to be discussing their mother leaving a place she had lived in since 1990.

They were probably thinking like me that once she left her home she would never return.

Chapter 21

It did prove to be extremely difficult to find anywhere suitable and local for the children. A new care home in our town had recently opened up but they only took the elderly with Dementia, and because of a few teething problems, they couldn't even contemplate a lady of forty-nine with Motor Neurone. I actually wondered if the teething problems were that the residents had been escaping and found wandering along the high street. This made me smile at the thought of little old men and women starting a tunnel like in the Great Escape. Of course it was disappointing that it wasn't to be, as being so close to home it would have been so easy to see Diana any time of the day and not rely on lifts all the time.

Two other homes were contacted but they also didn't have the facilities to cope with Motor Neurone and with Dementia on top of that. I looked on the Internet and reluctantly phoned a place called Beecher Hall. It had younger patients with difficult illnesses and the severely handicapped. If they agreed to consider Diana it would mean it was really going to happen. While homes were refusing it meant she stayed at home a little longer. We knew what was the best for her and for us but it was so hard letting go.

Beecher Hall was just a little further along from the Duchess of Kent. I spoke to the manager, a really friendly reassuring lady called Janet. She was very sympathetic to our problem and said if a room became available Diana could have it. She told me that they already had someone there with Motor Neurone; a man with a young family. He, unlike Diana, was in a wheelchair. He could still speak, but could not walk, the complete opposite to Diana. This disease held no prisoners; from the very start it altered your life, no drug could keep it at bay or slow up the symptoms.

Luckily Ali from the Primary Care Trust had already been in contact with Janet and had tried to phone me earlier in the day to explain her find. Janet told me that the funding had to be agreed and of course the one to one care. She told me that she couldn't see any reason for it to be refused and couldn't see any problem looking after Diana at the home.

This made me feel more positive. This lady knew her job and understood the kind of care we were looking for.

Janet asked if we would like to come and have a look round before any decisions were made.

I reluctantly with a heavy heart agreed to visit that weekend, almost hoping, I suppose, that I wouldn't like the place.

It was nothing like the Duchess of Kent. It was a very big place, it was carpeted with a dark blue patterned carpet that stretched along corridors that never seemed to end. I also noticed the place had a strange odour, I suppose it was inevitable in a place full of incredibly sick people that it would smell strange. This was a place where sick people ended their days. My heart started to thump in my chest realising this could be the place where my sister ended hers. She wouldn't understand why we were leaving her here; she would hate it but what choice did we have? She needed so much more now and my niece and nephew and the carers could no longer cope.

I wished it was more like the Duchess of Kent but it wasn't.

It was clean but so imposing because of its size.

There were three floors; the top floor homing the very disabled. We looked on all three floors. I noticed most bedroom doors stayed open, I couldn't help glancing in each of them as we passed by. People were either sat by their beds or laid quietly in them. Each room was different; they were very comfortable and had paintings on the walls and personal belongings making them very cosy. It was seeing the inside of these rooms that made me feel more positive. If Diana did come here we could make it cosy and like her home with a few of her own belongings just like all the other rooms I had seen. I know for a fact it didn't matter how nice the room was my sister's choice would have been to end her days in her own home, but that wasn't an option now. Liam and Lauren couldn't be subjected to more sleepless nights and exhausting days. Beecher Hall could give her what we couldn't any longer: round the clock specialist care. We were all mentally and physically exhausted.

The two children couldn't go on any longer, to get as far as they had was a miracle.

We left Beecher Hall feeling more positive but I felt very scared. I was dreading the day Diana would leave her home, getting into our car believing she was going for a drive, trusting us as she always did.

There was no point telling her our intentions. We could never have made her understand why we were sending her from her home and from her children. She would have been mortified if she had known how much the kids had to cope with. She would have been the first to agree that we had no other choice, and it was the right choice.

The funding was approved that following week. Jack phoned me to tell me the news, and also the one to one care as Diana could not be left on her own for a single minute.

This was now to be the hardest part of the last two and a half years. We all felt heavy hearted and my guilt was as high as it could be. I felt we were letting Diana down. Lauren and I packed her clothes the day before she was due at Beecher Hall. Diana didn't take any notice as we were always sorting out one thing or another. We emptied her drawers in complete silence just making the odd comment about what we should pack. If I felt bad how must Liam and Lauren feel? That night in bed I kept telling myself that it was the only choice we had. Diana was too poorly now to be at home, the carers were exhausted and couldn't cope any longer. They weren't trained for this terrible illness. The night staff could not keep Diana in her bed and Liam and Lauren were having hardly any sleep. Deep down it was right but it didn't make it any easier. I don't think I slept much that night, I couldn't even concentrate on the telly and the words in my book just jumbled together. In the end I came downstairs and made a cup of tea, wishing I could switch my brain off just to give me a bit of peace. Thinking is very tiring and I just couldn't stop thinking about my sister and what awaited us the next day. By morning I felt awful, my eyes were bloodshot from lack of sleep. I showered which woke me up a little. My stomach was churning over and I couldn't eat any breakfast. We went to collect Diana and Lauren at twelve p.m. My poor sister must have thought she was going for a ride in our car; the one thing she loved doing. She became anxious, moving from side to side as she couldn't wait for us to get her coat on and get in our car. Liam gave his mum a big hug; he didn't want to come with us as he couldn't cope with it. Luckily Rita came home for her lunch, she saw Liam at the front door sobbing and went to be with him while we drove away. This was Diana's final journey, away from her family, her beloved home and her neighbours. I wanted to cry and sob so badly but I couldn't. Lauren cuddled up to her mum; I put on the car radio as none of us felt like talking. Diana just stared out of the window unaware of our destination. I know they say you have to be cruel to be kind but this was the cruellest situation, and the cruellest disease. We could never show our emotions in front of her, she wouldn't understand why we cried it would make her cry. All I could think was, 'She's only forty-nine, why has this happened to a girl so full of life and only half way through it?!'

I will never know the answer and no one will ever have an explanation for it. And I will never accept it. I suppose it was just her time. What I don't understand is why Liam and Lauren should lose a father and then their mother. I don't think there will ever be a day I say, 'Ah, that's why it happened.'

They say as one door closes another one opens. Well let's wait and see shall we? It will have to be a big bloody door to make it up to Liam and Lauren.

As we pulled into the gravel drive at Beecher Hall Diana was still unaware of the situation. It wasn't until she saw a nurse come towards us as we entered the front door, that she stepped back and tried to pull away from Lauren's hand. She tugged at Lauren's arm, her face looked frightened and her feelings were very clear. Here she did not want to be!

How we managed the next hour I don't know. We were taken to Diana's room by a nurse, Diana kept stopping but had no choice but to come with us as we kept walking. The room, which was smaller than some of the ones we had peered into only the week previous, wasn't very appealing. It was frankly bland; a bed, a wardrobe, a chair, a dressing table, and an adjoining toilet. The bed took up all the room as it was stuck out in the middle of the room. I would have arranged it differently, putting the bed along the wall giving the room a bit more space. Lauren looked horrified. Her words were, 'This room is shit, we can't leave Mum here, she'll hate it, Aunty Jan.'

I didn't know how to respond, I agreed it wasn't the nicest of rooms but we needed to make it homely with Diana's own stuff; this I said to Lauren. Diana had already gone walkabout looking for a way out just as she had done at the Duchess of Kent. Luckily the nurse was already after Diana. She walked with her along the two long corridors that led from Diana's room. She was already planning her escape! I don't want to sound blasé about the situation but if I didn't try to look at the humorous side of things I truly believe one of us would have had a breakdown. My bet would have been Lauren.

'Lauren,' I said, 'I will go tomorrow and get your mum a painting for the wall and her own pillows. We can bring in her bits from home and the coloured blanket Grandma had crocheted would look lovely on your mum's bed. We can bring in a few of her ornaments and one of her lamps, also some fluffy cushions would look good in her armchair.'

Diana was nowhere to be seen as we made plans for this warm but whitewashed, cold-looking room.

Lauren had calmed down just as Janet the manager I had spoken to arrived to greet us. She also decided that the bed was in completely the wrong place and promised it would be moved the following day.

We decided to leave as soon as we had unpacked Diana's belongings as every time the nurse led her back she tugged at Lauren, pleading with her eyes to take her home. It felt so cruel, I felt like the most evil hardest person in the world. Right at this very moment I was the devil and I felt like it. It was no good trying to sit Diana down and explain everything to her. There was no reasoning left in her to understand why we were doing this. We had no other choice open to us.

Janet was very nice telling us that Diana would never be left on her own and we could ring or visit any time of the day. And we could change her room any way we wished.

So the next time Diana returned from walkabout Lauren kissed her mum, then I kissed her bony cheek with the biggest lump in my throat ever! As she turned away from the room again thinking we were following we went in a different direction. In fact we hid from her; there was no easy way of leaving her behind. I watched as she shuffled along the carpet, slowly one foot in front of the other, the nurse's arm through hers. My pathetically thin, indescribably sick sister was now at her final destination. And looking at her now I didn't think it would be for much longer, to carry on like this was the cruellest of the cruel. I cannot begin to describe how guilty I felt; ashamed, culpable, shameful, guilt-ridden, and a bad person. I was all these words and more. I had to get out, as to see her face again before we left was too much to bear.

In the car I kept talking to Lauren. We would make her mum's room comfy and bring in the things that she knew; I would go and buy her a nice painting to brighten the drab magnolia walls. Lauren then suggested she make a collage with family photos; she said she would use her own notice board hanging in her bedroom and cover it with all the family members and my new baby granddaughter, as Diana loved Rianne. Lauren's mood shifted from one of despair to someone with a purpose. This is how we got through things, a plan, a purpose, an idea. It wasn't much but it helped my niece and if we had a plan it made us feel better. We were doing positive things to make us feel we weren't neglecting Diana. In between, heart attacks and aneurysms and bladder cancers, for the last three years Diana had been the main focus. It now had to be a focus on things to get done away from the care home; things to take in to her, things to buy, extra clothing too for her to wear, when to visit, what days to visit.

Liam and Lauren would now live on their own. It would now become very different at their home; no more carers coming day and night. The hordes of medical visitors that came were now not needed, the house would seem eerily quiet.

It was now back to me, Mum, Adam, the rest of the family, Mary our friend and Rita.

The house was to be sold when Lauren reached eighteen, as the judge when it went to court had awarded their father the majority of the share, the rest going to Liam and Lauren. I don't know how it would have gone if Diana was to survive, but I think Liam having learning difficulties should have been taken into consideration. Lauren wanted to be a hairdresser, they were never going to be big earners, so in one and a half years' time a home had to be found for them both. This I wasn't even going to worry about. Having enough money for them to live on was the first thing to sort out, as all Diana's benefits would stop; they would now go towards the care home.

It was with a very heavy heart that I climbed into bed that night. As I lay staring into the dark, Adam already sleeping beside me, I thought of my sister. Was she walking up and down the corridors looking for us or looking for a way out? Was she frightened? I knew she wouldn't understand why we had deserted her again.

It took me a long time until I finally fell asleep. For the last two and a half years my sleep pattern was all over the place. Some days it was from sheer mental exhaustion that I collapsed into bed. Those were the nights when I wouldn't have heard an explosion I was so tired; then other nights I tossed and turned well into the early hours.

We decided not to visit until the Sunday so that Diana could settle in. Mum didn't feel well enough to come with us, she said she would hopefully come the next time. We had packed the car with her ornaments and blankets. I had brought a pretty picture of bright red flowers to hang in the room, a lamp belonging to Diana and Lauren's lovingly made photo collage. Around the edges of the collage she had fixed a long pink feather decoration to bring colours into her drab room. I had also purchased two comfortable fluffy cushions to use on the leather chair in her room.

Diana cried as soon as she saw us. Her nurse was with her, he introduced himself as Andrew. He explained that they changed shift every two hours and let Diana go virtually where she wanted to. Straight away she headed down the corridor towards the front door, hoping I'm sure we would follow. Andrew her nurse followed as we had work to do. Adam hung the picture above her bed which as promised had been moved to a much better position, then we hung Lauren's collage on the opposite wall so Diana could see it while sat in her bed. I fixed up her freeview box, another purchase of mine. I know that television wasn't that important to her anymore, but when we weren't about did she actually watch any? Hopefully the background noise was familiar and comforting. I wanted her room to be as home-like as possible even if that meant her telly was only background noise. The room looked quite cosy when we had finished. Lauren by now was walking up and down with her mother, I joined them. The nurse left us to have a bit of time on our own with her. Diana must have already done quite a bit of walking because people were waving to her from their rooms as we went past. She held up her good arm and waved back, it was really sweet to be a part of it. Already the other patients were used to Diana frequently going past them. I don't know how I felt about her being at Beecher Hall, it just felt good that we had the freedom to spend quality time with her. We didn't dress her or shower her anymore or have the awful trouble of getting her medicine into her, and we weren't constantly on edge. We had the best part, visiting, holding her hand and walking with her, knowing she was in safe hands. Leaving would always be hard, but they were precious moments for us knowing we wouldn't have her for much longer.

We left at five p.m. because it was teatime. The nurse led Diana to the dining room, she went quite happily shuffling along the carpet. We followed behind but continued on towards the exit as they entered the smart little room full of freshly laid tables. It was the best time to go because this had distracted Diana from the upset of us leaving her.

We decided to go back in a couple of days. This time Mum came with us; she felt well enough to visit. Diana cried as soon as she saw us; we hugged her and gathered in her little room. I had taken in a fold down deckchair so that we all had seats to sit on. We kept the conversation light. Her carer left us to be alone with her. As usual Diana turned to leave the room. It was now our turn to walk backwards and forwards along the two corridors. We waved as Diana did to patients sat in their rooms. Diana's routine never changed, I hadn't needed the deckchair after all, Diana wasn't planning on doing any sitting, so arm in arm we went back and forth. She took us to the front door just as she had at the Duchess of Kent; she stopped and looked at it for quite a while. Did she think? Was she still capable of that? She obviously knew it was the door that led outside, but she had lost the capability of letting us know what she wanted.

She stared at the door, like she was straining her mind to remember how to communicate what she wanted.

It was very sad that we couldn't open that door and let her be free. She was trapped in her own body and mind.

Arm in arm we turned her round and headed back to her room, where Mum and Adam were waiting for us. As we walked Diana into the room she first waved at Mum and then at Adam, as if they had just turned up. We stood with her while Lauren pointed out the photos on the collage. Diana lifted her weak arm and pointed at all our familiar faces. Lauren had filled the board with about fifty photos. The nurse had previously told us that Diana liked to look at them and would point out each familiar face to each carer on the various shifts.

All too soon it was time to leave so Lauren went to fetch Diana's carer who Diana quite happily walked along the corridor with. We followed but turned a different direction as we had previously done the last visit, so she wouldn't become upset.

The talk in the car was always about Diana; how she seemed, how we felt seeing her, how she looked. We were all definitely more relaxed as she was being looked after so well, it gave us all peace of mind. Lauren was definitely happier at her mum being at Beecher. Seeing the care she was being given made us all feel better about her being there.

If she wanted to walk up and down the corridors all day then that's what they let her do, they couldn't stop her anyway, as Diana was determined to continue her routine.

It was decided we would go again the next night. Mark my middle son wanted to visit, so he followed us to Beecher Hall. Liam also came; as I said once before he found his strength from his cousins and once he knew Mark was going that made up his mind.

Mark's face said it all when he set eyes on his aunty. He hadn't seen her for quite a few weeks; his shock was evident to see. Diana was seated in the communal sitting room with her carer. Even to me she seemed so much worse, her face was sallow and her chest rose higher than normal. She looked at Mark and his girlfriend with wide, scared eyes. I knew then that she didn't recognise them. Mark I could see was very upset, he left the room followed by Kylie his girlfriend and Liam. I was told later that he had sobbed outside in the car park. He couldn't believe how much she had changed in such a short while as the reality set in Diana did not have much longer to live.

When he returned to us he had composed himself. Diana looked at him and then she waved at him, she suddenly knew who he was.

'Yes, Diana,' I said, 'you know Mark.'

She nodded, then tried to get out of her chair, we were going walkabout again. Slowly we headed along the corridor, Lauren one side, me the other, passing the same open rooms as before, Diana waving as we passed.

Her body was so much frailer, her legs too weak and heavy now for her to move along the thick navy carpet without help. I prayed to myself that her suffering would soon end; it was killing me to see her like this. I felt such guilt that it was her and not me.

Her carer came to her room to be with her, the telly was showing *Eastenders*. We sat her in her big comfortable chair,

Diana didn't attempt to get up this time, the walk from the sitting room had obviously drained any strength she had left.

We sat with her for a while, Mark and kylie came to say goodnight, we followed on a little later.

We were all quiet in the car, Diana was different tonight; we had all noticed it but nobody mentioned it.

As I got into bed that night I had a feeling things were going to change. I was right. Early in the morning I got a phone call from Beecher Hall saying Diana was having difficulty breathing, and did I want them to ring an ambulance.

'Of course,' I snapped, 'my sister must not suffer.'

Then I went to pieces. I rang my mother in floods of tears.

'I don't know what to do.' I was crying hysterically. 'I can't cope, Mum.'

'Yes you can,' she said. 'Get dressed and we will go to the hospital, I'll ring Liam and Lauren,' she said.

I managed to calm down, as my niece and nephew needed strength not hysteria.

Liam decided he couldn't cope with seeing his mother as none of us knew what we would find at the hospital. He instead came over to stay with my daughter-in-law Chloe.

Heavy hearted we set off for the Royal Berks. We went to casualty as instructed; what greeted us was so very awful. Diana lay in a hospital bed, her eyelids half closed over her eyes, I could see she was in a coma. We stood there the three of us crying quietly. I held my sister's hand; Lauren stroked her forehead, and my mother stood looking at her youngest daughter she looked pale and so much older.

The doctor came into the little cubicle. He told us that Diana wasn't suffering and that because her breathing had become so bad the carbon dioxide we breathe out had entered her blood stream, this then puts the patient into a coma-like state.

I will be honest I expected to see her on oxygen struggling for every breath, but there she lay calm and peacefully breathing unaided, not suffering or struggling as I had anticipated at home. This was the time since Diana had been diagnosed that I had been dreading, but looking at her now I knew the end was finally near. She didn't deserve to die but she deserved to have an end to her suffering. I felt so scared. I had never seen anyone die before and now it was to be my own flesh and blood. She lay so perfectly still, her breathing was quiet. I kissed her forehead, which felt clammy and cold, and I whispered, 'You can go now, Diana, go and find peace and happiness, we'll be ok.'

The rest of my family were making their way in, John, Mark, James and also Liam. He had decided he wanted to come once he knew his cousins were coming. Also our friend Mary and her husband Ed and one of our favourite carers Amanda.

We were taken with Diana to a private room so that we could be with her undisturbed. A nurse asked if we would like a priest to come and say a prayer before everyone else arrived.

I agreed to her suggestion. Adam went to wait for the others while the three of us sat around her bed. The whole time Diana didn't move. The rise and fall of her chest and her shallow breaths were the only sound, it didn't seem appropriate to talk; it felt disrespectful to her.

The hospital priest was an older man with an accent; it felt calming to have him with us (no one else had arrived yet). He spoke softly and asked if we would like him to bless Diana and say a prayer. In turn he asked our names, then he began his prayers. As he spoke we lowered our heads and stood looking towards my sister. I held her hand as tears rolled down my cheeks. As he said his prayers I heard him say, 'I am here with your mother Margery, your sister Jan and your daughter Doreen'.

Well I nearly exploded; did he really call Lauren Doreen? Great, a deaf priest! He carried on with the prayer and then again he said, 'God bless Margery, God bless Jan and God bless Doreen.'

Well that did it for me. I couldn't look at my mum or Lauren. I let out a sort of snort which I then tried to disguise as a sob. My God, it always happened to us; something so poignant and serious and the priest gets my niece's name wrong. When he left we couldn't help it, we all started to giggle. I held Diana's hand and said to my mum, 'Diana would have laughed her head off at that.'

She would have found it so funny and I know she wouldn't have minded us laughing as she lay there. My sister had the best sense of humour, she would have been the first to join in.

Looking back there is no special way to behave; people cope in very different ways when it comes to a death.

One by one everyone that meant something to Diana came to be with her. All the people she cared about were in her room. We talked to her, we cried, we reminisced and we laughed. I really hope that she heard us and knew we were there. I already knew she wasn't suffering in that body anymore but maybe she was already looking down, as she passed from one life to the next.

At six o'clock that evening I could see my mum was exhausted. We had been with Diana since eight a.m. that morning. 'Why don't you go home, Mum? You look so tired.'

'I'll take you, Grandma,' John offered.

'Thank you, darling, my back is very bad,' she replied.

This next moment will stay with me forever. Our mother walked slowly to my sister's bed and leant forward. With tears in her eyes she said goodbye to her daughter. 'Goodbye, darling – see you soon.'

My brave mum was saying her last goodbye to her youngest child. It was the saddest moment I had ever experienced. No parent expects a child to go before they do, and as she walked away from the room there wasn't a dry eye between us.

We all sat quietly as we let the moment wash over us. I couldn't get it out of my mind and to this day it is one of the memories that stays with me.

One by one family and friends left, each in turn kissing Diana on her cheek, until it left me, Lauren and Adam. By now it was seven-thirty and I could see poor Lauren was shattered. Diana's breathing was still strong. I knew it was best to get Lauren home, but I had to make a decision and it frightened the hell out of me. Should I stay on my own until she passed away? As I thought about it I knew I couldn't. If Diana had been conscious I would have one hundred percent stayed with her to the end as I couldn't bear for her to be awake and terrified. But I knew I didn't have the courage to be there as she took her final breath. I knew I would go to pieces if I was there at the end. I could say I felt guilty now about not staying and that I had failed her but I had to do what was right for me, as I think it would have haunted me for the rest of my life.

I had never experienced death before, never expecting it to be someone so close to me, and it frightened the hell out of me.

I asked the nurse on duty if we could have a pair of scissors so that we could take a lock of her hair before we left and in turn we kissed her and said our goodbyes to her. The tears burned my eyes as we walked away knowing this was to be the last time I would see my special sister. The nurses were there with her.

We were all silent on the journey home. Lauren was having trouble keeping her eyes open and I stared into the dark taking notice of nothing.

I can honestly say that I slept very deep that night. I was mentally and physically exhausted and fell asleep as soon as my head hit the pillow.

At five-twenty that morning the phone went. I knew exactly who it would be. The nurse sadly told me Diana had very peacefully passed away at ten past five that morning and ironically, it was as I said at the beginning of my story, the day she had married twenty-eight years ago. 6th March 1982.

It was like she was waiting for that day, the day that had made her so happy. She had married Sean, lost him and then died on the day that had meant so much to her.

I lay back in bed it was no good ringing my mother or Liam and Lauren that early as there was nothing anyone could do. I felt so empty, so flat in fact I really don't know how I felt; relieved, exhausted, numb. It all felt so unreal; this wasn't my life it was someone else's. I couldn't cry, I was all cried out.

I think relieved more than anything as her suffering was at an end.

All of us spending that time with her was so uplifting, I'm so glad we said our goodbyes. The people that stayed true to Diana, not the others and they know who they are, who never wrote to her when she was deserted. Especially the people she had regarded as her best friends, who she went to school with and then worked with, not a note a phone call or a visit. But all through her hurt and pain she never said a bad word about anyone.

She always hoped Sean would come back, that is until her Dementia made her forget him. I thank God for that.

Chapter 22

The next few days were like being on auto pilot; Diana had died but it didn't seem real.

We all hugged as we met, all of us relieved that it was finally over. Diana at last was with her maker, and an angel to watch over her children.

We carried on as normal as we could that day as shopping had to be done, so we made our weekly trip to Lidl as we always had. Liam didn't come with us preferring to be with his friends; Lauren as usual came with us. To be honest it didn't seem real. I think we felt in limbo; how do you behave? What do you do? Only the silence at their home made it real.

Later that day Adam phoned the funeral directors on my behalf, and with their direction told us what needed to be done. We were given an appointment for Monday and everything would be explained from there.

Mum, Adam and I spent all the weekend with Liam and Lauren only leaving them to return to our beds. We talked about Diana and reminisced, we cried, we tidied and did washing and carried on as normally as we could. In the evening we discussed the funeral, how we wanted it and which song to be played at the end of the funeral. I had heard one sung by Leona Lewis called *run*, if you listen to the words and the music it is a beautiful song choice for a funeral.

I played it to our gathering, Liam, Lauren, James, myself and Adam. Mum had already gone home as, poor thing, she looked shattered. We sat listening to it in total silence. It says so much so perfectly. Of course we all had tears rolling down our cheeks by the end of it. It may sound strange that we weren't all sat huddled in despair in no condition to function, but arranging a funeral takes a lot of thought and careful decisions. Life has to go on. Diana was at peace now which is what we had wanted for a while. Listening to the song and talking about all we had dealt with helped us to release our emotions and it gave us yet another plan to work on. It was better for Liam and Lauren to keep occupied. I had my sister to say goodbye to and I wanted her day to be the best and remembered by everyone that attended it.

I wanted everything to be perfect. Diana's illness had ravaged her body and her looks, I wanted people to see how beautiful my sister was, so I chose a picture of Diana when she had been my bridesmaid at my first wedding. She was only eighteen but she was stunning, it was already quite a large photo so I knew I could get it made a lot bigger without it blurring.

When Monday came it was with a heavy heart that Adam and I collected Lauren then my mother, and made our way to the funeral directors. We were greeted by a young girl called Helen who explained things and made everything so much easier for us. They would take care of the printing for the service booklet, we had to decide which hymns we would like, also they would arrange for the vicar to ring me and meet us all.

I gave Helen a poem I had written which I asked to be printed in the service book.

> Now my soul has been set free
> Please don't sit and cry for me
> Miss me a little, then dry your tears
> My love surrounds you, I'm still here
> Though you may not see my face
> Look for me I'm every place
> I'll call to you through winds that blow
> I'll walk beside you wherever you go
> Still speak to me and I will hear
> I'm not gone, I'm somewhere near.

Lauren had chosen a picture of her mother to be printed on the front of the service booklet; a picture of Diana when she was in her thirties and just as lovely with her big beautiful smile. I had already decided to write something about Diana as a tribute to her, I just had to make sure everything I said was perfect.

We chose a dark wood coffin and asked for the flowers to say Mother, Daughter and Sister.

Adam had taken a couple of days off work as the next day we had to go to the hospital to collect a document called a green slip so that her body could be released to the care of the funeral directors. Then we had an appointment at two o'clock so that we could register the death and collect the death certificate.

We went in to automatic again, not really quite believing that this was happening. I sort of shut my mind down trying not to think of Diana, and that all we were doing was for another person, another Diana not our Diana. She was still at the care home still walking up and down the two long corridors. But in the back of my mind I was dreading the day when the hearse containing her coffin arrived at the front of the house. I tried not to think about it, I had to blank my mind as it hurt like hell when I did.

I wrote my piece about Diana as I lay in bed. I always managed to think clearer there and of course it was where I did my worrying. I read it to my youngest son, I told him I would find it very hard to read. 'I'll do it, Mum,' he said.

Well I was quite shocked but really touched that he had offered as James can be quiet. If anyone it would have been John that I would have bet on. He could sell snow to the Eskimos and holds no fear standing up and speaking on my behalf.

'Are you sure, James? You will need to read it loud and clear.'

With that he held the piece of paper and very clearly and with his voice raised, he read my piece out perfectly. I felt very proud that he should offer to read it on my behalf, although I know either of his brothers would have also done so.

The next thing was to choose a date for the funeral; the date decided was to be Thursday, 18th March. It gave us enough time to let people know about Diana and it gave us a bit of breathing time. The Vicar had arranged to come and see us on the Tuesday the week before the funeral.

She was young and very pleasant. She explained everything to us, going through each part of the service; the prayers, the hymns, in what order etc. Then she wanted to know about Diana. In turn we all said our bit about her, Lauren Liam, myself and Mum. Marion (her name) said that it would be very upsetting as the reality finally hits you; it is the last part of Diana's and your incredible and painful journey, but that it was also a celebration of Diana's life and a way to say your goodbyes.

Marion had already left me an order of service, which I said was fine, it just had to be agreed when James should read on my behalf; it was decided after the first hymn. And Run would be played at the end of the service, Marion would read my poem after she had spoken about Diana. I felt relieved when everything was finally in place. The next day Helen phoned me from the funeral directors; they needed to know if we wanted Diana dressed in anything special, I told her I would speak to Lauren first.

Diana liked the colour turquoise and some of her clothes were in that colour. It had also suited her complexion so we chose a turquoise checked top that I had got for her in the summer and a beautiful turquoise cardigan and her black trousers. Lauren also wanted her fluffy dog she had brought for her mother to be included in her coffin.

Marion had also said if we wanted to write any notes these could be placed on the coffin as she said the final prayers.

The next day I took the clothing and the CD I had recorded with the music on and gave them to Helen. I thanked her for making life a little easier.

Chloe came up with a good idea of us wearing turquoise accessories. Diana liked the colour and had quite a few items of clothing in this colour. It would be as a mark of respect and the boys, John, Mark, James and Liam would wear matching turquoise ties. They were to carry the coffin, a very brave thing to do I thought. I felt so proud of them all and so would Diana.

This again was another plan to keep Liam and Lauren busy. Lauren wanted to go and buy turquoise jewellery and they also wanted to write a private note from her and Liam. I gave her a notelet and envelope. I also wanted to write something not the same as James was reading but something more personal from me to Diana. I cried as I wrote as it was so difficult saying goodbye to my sister.

Even to this day I still can't believe she's not with us. Being busy and occupied does help. It's the quiet days that I find myself thinking about her. It's never the sick Diana, it is the well Diana; the giggly, generous one. Certain things come to my mind, sometimes it's when we were kids, but mostly it's the times involving our children when they all played together in Diana's back garden, while we sat drinking tea watching them play.

Some days I feel so angry as she loved her life, and looked forward to special events like Christmas, the Pantomime we never missed, Easter, her holidays, meeting up with our friends once a week for our animated chats. An outsider listening in would have been bored but we thrashed out who should go through in X-factor, and who was annoying us in I'm a Celebrity, we'd laugh at my cooking disasters, the state of the country and so on.

We would go in to town together a few times a month on the bus and we always went in at Christmas to buy presents and then back on the bus by lunchtime.

Once people knew of Diana's passing sympathy cards started to arrive through the letter box. At first I didn't find them comforting, just another reminder that Diana wasn't here anymore. I couldn't read the words; just a quick glance at who the card was from then I left them face down on the breakfast bar.

It is natural and kind to send condolences to friends and loved ones I know that, but it doesn't help initially; not for a little while anyway, the hurt needs to die a little. I was then able to sit in the quiet and read each one and the beautiful words that then can lift your spirit and give you hope. That is when I felt able to put them on display.

Chapter 23

Diana's Funeral

The day of the Funeral arrived. I felt sick to my stomach as soon as I opened my eyes from a very difficult sleep. I couldn't eat my usual piece of toast for breakfast, I just about managed to drink a cup of tea, I had a nervous stomach so I visited the loo several times during the morning.

Eventually it was time to gather at Diana's house. The boys looked very smart with their turquoise ties and the girls and myself wore turquoise jewellery and Lauren and I had painted our finger nails turquoise to match.

Making conversation was difficult. What could we possibly talk about while waiting for the hearse to arrive? I was feeling physically sick by now.

'The cars are here, Mum,' one of the boys called.

Slowly each one of us walked outside. It was freezing cold and the wind was blowing but the sun was out. My face felt flushed and I could feel my rapid heartbeat against my ribcage. I looked up and there it was, the large, black, shiny hearse. The first thing I saw were the flowers saying 'Sister' lying against Diana's coffin. All the pain, all the hurt rushed at me. This was the moment it hit me, as I knew it would. The moment I was dreading, seeing her coffin, the reality hit me like a cannonball. Tears rolled down my face and my dad started to sob, Mum was dabbing her eyes with her hanky and poor Lauren started to shake uncontrollably, tears also falling down her cheeks.

The day I had been dreading since Diana's diagnosis was finally here. It would have been so easy at that moment to run away and never come back.

The last piece of the journey had started, the lump in my throat hurt like hell as I tried to stop my sobs.

The boys went to their cars; Liam chose to go with James and not in the funeral car with us. Adam sat in front with Lauren while I sat next to Mum and Dad in the back.

The journey to the crematorium wasn't very far but it seemed to take forever as of course out of respect the car travels at a slow pace. We followed the hearse but I couldn't look at it, it was hard to see the coffin knowing it held my sister's body. I looked out of the side window whilst trying to calm down my racing heart and clear the painful lump in my throat. I had been dreading this day since Diana had been diagnosed and now it was here.

Please, God, help me cope!

Quite a few people were stood waiting outside the neat little Chapel as our cars pulled up. And bless her heart even though she had been unwell for a while my mother-in-law Beth had come all the way from Dorset with Adam's sister Sarah and husband Rob travelling about a hundred and twenty miles to be with us.

The Vicar Marian stood to one side of the entrance to allow people in as it was freezing stood outside; we were to follow behind the coffin. Marion said to wait a while just in case any people were late.

Poor Lauren still shook uncontrollably; Mum put her arm around her shoulders, as the wind was so bitterly cold. I couldn't feel a thing, shock I think, I just wanted to get in and be seated.

Finally the pallbearer beckoned the boys over and instructed them how the coffin should be held. That moment will stay with me also. I felt such pride that they should wish to do this for their aunty and Liam for his mother.

Slowly we walked behind, Mum next to Lauren, me next to Dad holding his arm to steady him and Adam just behind us. My life suddenly flashed before me: we were children again running around the garden laughing out loud, without a care in the world, then mothers sharing our days with our children. And now here I was following her coffin holding the body of my beloved sister. My sister whom God chose to take at the age of forty-nine.

How I managed to walk behind her coffin I don't know; my legs felt like they would buckle any moment. I kept my head bent towards the floor, I couldn't look to the front and see the faces looking sad for her and for us. The tears blurred my vision, I didn't look up, but straight at the floor.

I sat down in between Dad and Lauren and then took a quick glance about me. The chapel was packed, I was so pleased to see how many people had come to say goodbye to Diana.

The beautiful photograph of her was placed at the front of the chapel on a table for all to see.

The service was as I had hoped it would be, it was beautiful and unforgettable. Marion said lovely things about Diana, and James read loudly and clearly as I had requested, he didn't let me down, his voice started to crack at the end but he cleared his throat and got there.

The poem I wrote Diana, Marion read out for me. I knew I couldn't do it. I wanted something personal in the service booklet.

I could hear a few sobs behind me, and my dad sobbed quietly as he listened.

Marian then asked if anyone would like to come and stand by the coffin while she said a prayer. Lauren and I left our seats both clutching the notes we had written, then alongside us came Mary, the three of us placed our hands on the coffin. Lauren and I then placed our notes on the top; poor Lauren still shook the whole time. But so brave.

I could hear Marion's voice but I couldn't take in what she was saying, I was only aware of the soft shiny wood under my cold hands knowing that next to me lay my sister's body, just wood between us; so near but so far. I put my head near to the wood and whispered goodbye to her.

We went back to our seats and sang the final hymn. I could hear sniffing and quiet crying behind me it was such an emotional service, but it went exactly how I had wanted it to.

Marian's words brought her back to us for a little while, surrounded by those who meant a lot to her, the people that mattered. The ones that gave up on her stayed away, what they believed and what they were made to believe was up to them. Knowing her for so long didn't seem to make a difference; even a card to Liam and Lauren just to show that they cared would have been something. Liam and Lauren had a right to feel angry and hurt with family members, their father had walked out and their mother had died, stories were told and believed. With all that has happened they need stability and to know that it's ok to feel hurt and be angry and cry and miss their mum and not be judged if they decide not to see their father. I go along with their wishes. If one day they want to make contact it is fine by me; my life goes on regardless.

But sides are always taken in a break-up and subsequent divorce and it is always the kids that suffer.

No sooner had the service begun it was over, the doors were opened and the beautiful voice of Leona Lewis filled the chapel.

Slowly one by one we left, I cannot write about the curtains closing around Diana's coffin it is far too painful.

Outside the cold wind revived me as my face felt hot and flushed, inside I was still shaking.

One by one I went to every little group to thank them for coming; some still had tears in their eyes as Leona Lewis's voice drifted to the outdoors. They all said the same thing, 'What a beautiful funeral it had been.'

Back at the house Amanda, Katherine and Hayley the nurse, took charge of making the tea, which was a relief. It was nice just to sit and unwind. The immediate family were exhausted.

I thanked my mother-in-law Beth for making the long journey, it was nice to sit and chat to the friends and neighbours who had come back to the house. Lauren was much better now and had stopped shaking, and I could tell she was enjoying having a packed house, and having the two favourite carers and mad Hayley the Scottish nurse made the atmosphere light.

I still couldn't eat a thing but managed a cup of tea; I talked in turn to the various people that had come back to be with us.

I used to wonder how people could invite people back to their homes after a funeral. Tradition or not it seemed strange to be in despair one minute then eating sandwiches with the crusts cut off the next, but now I know – it felt comforting to talk and be surrounded by people who cared and could take over for a bit, and if you didn't want to talk you could sit and listen. I finally managed to eat one sandwich just to take away my sick feeling as I hadn't eaten all day. Not once did I feel like asking people to leave.

I remember thinking Diana would have loved this. She liked a get together.

When I climbed into bed that night of course I lay thinking about the day. I felt so proud that Liam and Lauren had been so brave and that Liam and the boys had carried her coffin, their very last bit of contact with Diana, to safely deliver her to her maker.

As a family we had taken care of all her needs, apart from some of her care that she had to have from nurses etc., we didn't and couldn't have physically coped twenty-four-seven. Every decision we made as a family and were always in Diana's best interest.

We probably made wrong decisions and lost our tempers but all in all I think we did our best for Diana especially for her children. Rest in peace, my beloved sister.

Chapter 24

After the funeral we all felt deflated, so being busy was the best thing to keep our minds occupied. Money had to be sorted, people had to be notified about Diana's death, her bank account had to be closed, so even if we needed a breather it wasn't going to be for a while.

Diana's benefits would stop so now there would only be Liam's Disability Living Allowance coming in.

Lauren didn't want to stay on for further education as she had missed so much school in the last year it would be impossible to catch up on all she had missed.

She had always wanted to be a hairdresser so we found her a job; thanks to John's friend Eddie for speaking to his boss the owner of the hairdressing salon 'Julian's'. She has taken to it like a duck to water and is attending college once a month; Mondays are her training day and like her mother was in her job, Lauren has become a very popular member of the hairdressing team.

Life goes on for us all. We have bad days and good days.

I had to go the doctors after Diana died as my mood was very low and with so much still to do I knew I needed help. I had become very panicky when I had to go anywhere especially with others in our car. I can't explain why that was, I knew the signs and the feelings and had to try and nip it in the bud. It just panicked me one day and I found myself making excuses not to be in the car if anyone requested a lift. Liam still needed help and had been requested to attend meetings concerning his benefits, Mum was due for her check-up, I knew that even though Diana had gone I would still have so much to do. I would never turn my back, but coping with anxiety and feeling panicky is very difficult to ignore when so much around you is going on. My doctor put me on an anti-depressant and suggested I be seen by talking therapys; therapy by talking over the phone at an agreed time. I will say that it didn't really help me (the talking bit); the medication was my saviour, the counsellor was nice but it was as I knew it would be: I had to deal with my demons, no one could do it but me, but I needed my mood lifted before that could happen, without it I would never have coped. I tend to tell myself, 'You can do this,' even if I get stressed or panicky. I don't have the option to walk away, otherwise I am letting people down that need help. There was no one else to go with Mum or go with Diana or Liam.

Now Liam and Lauren were living on their own it was definitely much quieter. In fact at first they found it too quiet, the house, once crowded and hectic, was now eerily quiet. Lauren said they felt like orphans. This made me feel very sad for them. I assured them both I would always be there as long as they needed me. Mum and I still went round frequently to help with household chores as it was difficult for them to become motivated with cooking and cleaning etc. Lauren had her work which tired her out, stood on her feet all day, rushing around the hairdressers doing the menial tasks as apprentices do.

And Liam bless him, he tried hard but without a job he had nothing to get up for. I mean what boy would think about the dinner or the washing and the cleaning? Especially a boy with learning difficulties. They began to argue and then ring me up to come over as they became bored with each other's company. So now we have a good routine. Mum and I go over every week when we can to help out, cook dinner and do the ironing etc. They come to me a few evenings a week and over the weekend, usually Saturday and Sunday evening and I give them a dinner once a week, maybe more if I'm not too busy. (It is very difficult to have time to myself to write this.) We all meet on a Wednesday for our get together and Lauren calls in most days after work. They spend time with Chloe, and Lauren has been out a few times with James's new girlfriend Louise. They both have a good selection of friends. It needed time for the adjustment to their new way of life, but incredibly they are swimming not sinking. As Rita said the other day, they are both quite remarkable.

They have had a couple of bar-b-cues for their friends and behaved very well with no complaints from the neighbours and music was sensibly turned down before midnight.

They have days when everything hits them; one gets down and just needs a chat and a bit of company. Then the other has a bad day and needs the same reassurance.

Time I know heals, but to lose your mum so young will be something that stays with them forever.

They are a credit to their mother; I know she would be proud of them and the way they have handled the last few years.

One event that was fast approaching was Lauren's school prom; the first problem to solve was her dress, her shoes, and not having much money to purchase these items. And knowing the cost and affording a prom dress was going to prove difficult, until my daughter-in-law Chloe made the suggestion that the family club together and buy her the dress, shoes and accessories. It was the best idea we had.

It was agreed that each couple give £50, this then would at least give her enough to buy something she really liked and not something she had to settle for.

Of course she was so excited and over whelmed, as I know the prom, the expense and what to wear had been worrying her.

Her hair would not be a problem or an expense as her work colleagues were to do it for her on the day of the prom. They had already had a trial run on the style that suited her. Everything sorted; now it was time to go forth and find this special dress. Having boys, I had not experienced the mad frenzy and panic of finding the one!! The dress that no one else would be wearing, the colour, the style, the length, where to shop for it, so many important decisions and luckily for me Chloe and Kylie volunteered to be the shoppers to accompany Lauren. They were nearer her age and shopped more than I did. I hated shopping and wore baggy clothes to hide lumps and bumps and had no ideas on prom dresses.

I was getting off lightly!

The story told back to me after the epic shopping trip was a tale of hundreds of dresses tried on, nearly the one but not quite the one, a different shop then back to a shop already visited, only to start again somewhere else. Oh how glad am I that I didn't go, my feet and patience wouldn't have stood it.

The choice eventually made by Lauren was stunning. It took a while to find as was expected, but it was beautiful and she looked beautiful in it. A long off the shoulder floating chiffon in a deep salmon colour and silver shoes and clutch bag to match. It was perfect and the look on her face said it all, she truly looked so very happy and grown up.

At that precise thought I felt deeply sad, sad that her mother wasn't here to witness this, or to help choose the dress. Life was so unfair sometimes, I hoped that her mother was looking down and feeling proud of her beautiful daughter.

I remember how I felt seeing my three sons in their suits before their proms, so proud and aware that they were now young men, as Lauren was now a young lady.

I would have gladly given my right arm for Diana to be here to experience this (Bitch disease!)

And again I was thinking, 'Why?' but the answer never comes and it never will.

What I am now about to write is quite unbelievable, I'm still not sure how and what I feel about the following events.

The day of Lauren's prom arrived, luckily a lovely warm sunny June day; a perfect prom day.

Lauren was to have her hair done and then go to her friends to get ready. Mum, me and Adam were then going to her friends to see them leave in the vintage car that they had booked to take them to the school. We collected mum at seven and made our way to Lauren's friend's house. In my bag I had a disposable camera.

Both girls looked stunning and Lauren looked so very grown up, I felt tears well in my eyes but brushed them away as I gave her a hug; my thoughts were of Diana and how proud she would have been to see her daughter blossom into a gorgeous young woman.

I had given the camera to Adam as he took better photos than I did; I wanted the whole film used just for this occasion as a school prom is a big thing especially for a girl. He used the whole film on various shots, next to the car, in the car, on the lawn, by the front door, together and on their own. Every pose possible, they did it. Mum had been invited to stand just inside the house as it was incredibly hot and muggy. I was stood next to our car watching the chatting giggly girls and the posing they were doing for the cameras and loving every minute of it. Mum suddenly appeared from the door and hurried over to me and began to sob on my shoulder. This was the first time in my whole life I had ever witnessed my mother cry. She never cried, well properly cry, as she called it. She always said she couldn't cry but just got a lump in her throat. But here she was sobbing on my shoulder while I cuddled her. Lauren was too far away and luckily too pre-occupied to notice. It would have upset her to see her grandma so upset.

I got mum into the car while she pulled herself together. Lauren and her friend had seated themselves into the vintage car to take the customary ride through the streets before arriving at the school. They waved to us as they left, Lauren looking the happiest I had seen her in a while. Mum waved from the backseat with the window down.

'I don't know what came over me,' she said. 'I felt so strange, I couldn't stop crying.'

I told her that seeing Lauren so grown up and Diana not being there to see Lauren was too much for her to cope with.

'But I feel fine now. I just felt so weird. I couldn't control my emotions and I couldn't stop the tears.'

'Mum, don't worry it probably did you good to have a good cry, even though I have never in my life seen you sob.'

We took her home and went in with her for a cup of tea and a chat; she seemed ok so it wasn't mentioned again, not until a few days later that is.

We had taken the film to be developed the next day and told that the photos would be ready after the weekend, so Adam arranged to collect them as soon as he had finished work on the Tuesday.

He gave them straight to me as he came in. One by one I looked at them taking in every shot and detail as they had come out so perfectly. As I looked at one of the shots of the girls stood smiling by the front door, there looking from out of the doorway was the face of my sister, her smile, her hair style. My mum's skirt and part of her sunglasses were also visible and also the arm and checked top of Claire's mum. At first I thought I was seeing things and that it must be the face of Claire's mum, but the face I was looking at looked nothing like her mum. It was definitely the face of my sister looking out at her daughter. The funny thing is it didn't freak me out or give me goose bumps it made me feel strangely excited and happy. There she was looking straight at Lauren. Was that why mum had felt so emotional? Was that the precise time my sister had appeared next to her mother? I would have bet my house it was. I believe in life after death and seeing her didn't faze me one little bit. I called James and Adam to take a look, they both agreed that we were looking at the face of Diana. Liam and Lauren were coming over. I decided not to tell them, I wanted to see if they could see the same as us.

One by one Lauren went through the pictures then screamed, 'There's Mum, oh my God, oh my God.'

With that she burst into tears. By now John had turned up. At first he wasn't sure he agreed the face looked like Diana, but he queried what Claire's mum had looked like and was it a trick of the camera, or a shadow? I assured him that Claire's mum looked nothing like Diana and I told him what had happened to my mother at the same time.

John usually has to analyse everything which isn't a bad thing. As a child he was the same. 'But why? But where? But who? But when?' Question after question as he was doing now. I have always felt John would have made a good interrogator for the KGB or CIA as he questions everything and then can convince you, you are totally wrong when you know you are totally right. He wanted to know everything: where Grandma was stood, was there a photo of Claire's mum he could look at? Which luckily there was as he would have made my next mission to go and secretly photograph her so he could study her face. Never a dull moment with John around.

Lauren by now was animated, she was so convinced that her mother had been there and the effect it had on her and Liam was amazing. Like me it made them feel happy and in total agreement it was their mother.

We showed Rita the neighbour who had no doubt that she was looking at the face of Diana. I also showed Mandy our hairdresser when she next came, she had also previously cut Diana's hair. I didn't tell her what she was looking at. As I handed her the photograph she spotted Diana right away. 'Is that the last photo of Diana you have?'

'Mandy,' I said, 'Diana died in March. This picture was taken this June.'

'Oh my gawd, I've got goose bumps up and down my arm. I can't believe what I am seeing but there she is looking out at Lauren. I can't believe it but there she is.' Mandy had tears in her eyes. Seeing it had really affected her.

We discussed the photo while Mandy cut our hair, going over every possible scenario as to how she could possibly be in the photo and always reaching the same conclusion. The picture didn't lie; there she was in black and white or rather colour. Was it Diana letting her children know that she was watching over them?

I have always believed in life after death, ghosts and the paranormal so it really hadn't fazed me to see her there. It just confirmed my beliefs even more.

I still pick it up from time to time just to study the shot and to make sure she is still there.

A picture of my deceased sister captured on a photograph. Believe or don't believe that is a person's choice. John is still not convinced it is his aunty. Everyone else that has seen it feels the same as I do. It is Diana. I believe what I see and I am certain that it is Diana's way of confirming that there is something else out there.

My own experiences since living in my own home have made me absolutely sure that there is something on the other side. Of what, that I don't know, but life after death? It seems possible. I don't think my house is haunted but there have been a few instances that I cannot explain and a few I think I can. The first one was when John and Mark were about five and seven. It was very late at night, I was woken from my sleep by Mark. Very sleepily he told me that the bunk beds in which they slept in were rocking and it had woken him up. Without thinking about what he said and I suppose assuming he had been dreaming, I reluctantly got out of my warm bed and followed him sleepily into the room. Now bearing in mind these beds were solid metal and very sturdy, the bunk beds were indeed rocking side to side and it was quite pronounced as they swayed back and forth. In my half sleep state I stopped them and told Mark to get back into bed. I wandered back to my room; that's when it hit me and I fully woke up. 'My God, the bed was rocking,' I said out loud. I rushed back through. The bed was as I had left it still and rock solid, and Mark was now back, fast asleep. I know I didn't imagine it and Mark is usually a very deep sleeper so something woke him up. And I had stopped it from rocking; I had felt it move under my hands. John slept through it all. Good thing really as he would have been asking questions that I didn't have the answers to. I tried to rock the bed myself but it wouldn't budge because as I said it was solid metal and rigid. I have no explanation for that night. Mark remembered it in the morning but I made light of it by saying it was probably vibrations from heavy traffic. I didn't dwell on it so as not to frighten them. It never happened again and luckily it didn't seem to upset Mark. However it was something to tell my friends at our coffee mornings. Unnerve me? No. Puzzle me? Yes!

John and myself have both seen what we think is a young child; John will probably dismiss it now as he doesn't believe in ghosts. 'You die and that's it,' he announces if I tell the story. We were all in bed one night. James was about six and had climbed into bed with me and Adam as he always did if he woke out of a sleep. I heard John talking in the bedroom next to ours. 'Who are you talking to, John'? I called.

'James,' he replied (his room was in darkness).

'But James is in here with us,' I called back. With that John charged into our room switching on the overhead light blinding the three of us.

'Oh my God, I saw the figure of a boy about James's height stood at the end of my bed, I thought it was James and I was telling him to go back to bed.'

Again no explanation. Although John would now say he had probably been dreaming I feel differently.

I too have seen a young boy. Twice! Something woke me from a sleep and as I opened my eyes I saw the shape of a child next to me on the bed climbing up as if using stairs then disappearing through the wall. I screamed out and switched on the light. Poor Adam has been woken up so many times by me sleep talking, or sleep screaming, or not being able to sleep, turning the light back on to read and now I was seeing things and screaming out. He then jumped out of his skin thinking we were being attacked.

When Mark was about fifteen he had gone to bed early one night to use a sunlamp I had purchased years previously. It was to help John when he had suffered with bad spots. Mark by now had only a few blemishes, but enough to annoy him. I went in to say goodnight. He had on the protective goggles and had set the dial for ten minutes, it then switches itself off.

He was wide awake watching T.V. when I left his room.

I had fallen asleep pretty quick, and I dreamt. I don't remember the whole dream but it was about fire and burning. It woke me up with a start. It made no sense but I knew it meant something and I had to check on Mark and the sunlamp. I entered his room, I could hear the click click of the dial winding down on the sun lamp. Mark had fallen asleep, the dial had got stuck so the lamp was still on and still set at ten minutes and was shining onto his face which looked quite red. I woke him up immediately and warned him not use it again in bed as the dial had stuck, and he could have been badly burned. Again a mystery. Was the dream put there by his guardian angel to wake me up? Was it his guardian angel protecting him and waking me or was it my subconscious warning me, as that was the last thing in my head as I went to sleep? Always eventful in our house especially at night!

These three happenings I can't explain. The next two I feel were a hundred percent real. The first happened during Diana's illness; my stress levels were so high I was running on empty and knew that my depression was rearing its head again and I was feeling very agitated. I had been tossing and turning in bed for ages thinking about and worrying about everything that was happening to us as a family, truly not understanding why. It must have been the early hours. As I turned my head yet again towards my chest of drawers there at the side of me inches from the bed was a large white glow. Inside the glow was a child. It was so clear I could have reached out and touched his hand. It was a boy because he had short hair and was wearing shorts. The child stood to his side looking at me his head slightly lowered and to the side looking straight at me with a look of sympathy, maybe reassurance I don't know, definitely not hostile. He wore a shirt and shorts (the child I saw before this although only a dark outline also wore shorts). I lifted my head in disbelief and I again screamed, (think of poor Adam!) I switched on the light and looked about me. The glow and the child had gone, not surprisingly, this time I hadn't been woken from a sleep as I hadn't been able to sleep. I know what I saw, but it didn't freak me out, only the initial sighting.

What it meant I didn't know. I wish I hadn't screamed but it was a shock to see this child stood so close.

Only a few days earlier my mother had given me a clipping from the newspaper about people and their ghostly experiences with the same sort of thing and it stated that guardian angels appear as children because it is less frightening, (not so sure about that!) They can appear to you in times of great stress.

John called in the next morning. I called to him from the landing telling him what had happened. James who was still in his room came out as he heard what I was saying. He told me that he had woken up and had seen the white glow in his room next to the wall adjacent to mine (but not the figure). I at that moment knew a hundred percent I had not been dreaming. I was awake and I felt sure it was my guardian angel trying to reassure me that everything would be ok and that I would cope. It actually gave me a sense of peace and the courage and faith to go on and deal with things day by day. I felt I was being told that I was being looked after and that I would be ok. And not crumble as I feared.

The next event took place after Diana had died James had been unwell and was waiting for a hospital appointment, his life was on hold and he was extremely worried about his forthcoming diagnosis

He was suddenly woken out of a sleep, but he couldn't move, he felt someone holding his hand. He could feel their touch against his. It felt warm and the figure he saw in the dark he is convinced was the figure of my sister, his aunty. As she stood over him he couldn't breathe and he couldn't move. He said he felt frozen and knew if he tried he wouldn't have been able to, hence the saying frozen with fear! Not until she let go of his hand and then she disappeared. I am convinced she came to reassure him that he too would be ok and not to worry about his illness anymore. Since then Mum gave me a second hand book written by the healer Doris Stokes. She had helped Glen Hoddle and the England football team in preparation for the world cup, and also wrote of her experiences and why she became a healer. In one part she writes about a similar experience for a lady she was helping. They too had woken and found they couldn't move or get their breath until the vision left the room. James feels the same as I do, he had experienced exactly the same thing. John of course went down the who? Why? What? Where?

I have never felt uneasy in my home and my two dogs have never shown any distress at entering any of our rooms. Dogs are so aware of things around them, if they feel ok then so do I.

Chapter 25

Mum unfortunately it was decided had to have radiation treatment, which started in June for twenty-one treatments.

Again I started to feel panicky at the thought of going every day to the hospital. I had booked a few lifts with the cancer care trust then some with the hospital transport. I can honestly say I don't know how I got into the car that first day, my heart was racing and I was hot and clammy, but I hid it very well. I chatted away like a mad fool; this was to take my mind off of myself, I just couldn't let up with the chatter. I'm sure our driver thought I was the friendliest person in the world unaware of the panic I was feeling. When we arrived at the hospital I felt exhausted but also happy that I had made it in one piece without humiliating myself. The journey back was different again; don't ask me why. I suppose it was because I was going home, my sanctuary, my safe place. But the next day I felt the same again. This time we had a different driver and because of his age (most drivers are retired and volunteer workers) he drove very cautiously and announced we would go the slower, longer way as he wasn't keen on the motorway. Well that just about did it for me. Slower meant taking longer; I just wanted to get there. I think these people are marvellous giving up their free time to help people like my mother and in normal circumstances it wouldn't have mattered to me how fast we went but at present I was not coping very well.

Maybe God took pity on me or my guardian angel stepped in. James had not found his new job very easy, it just didn't suit him; it wasn't the big career change he thought it would be so he left right away. He had also started having more trouble with his what we thought was IBS. He started looking for something else. So he volunteered for a bit of petrol money to take my mother and I on days that he was free. So did my friend Mary, and Adam had already booked the last week off. My saviours! Not that they knew it apart from Adam that was.

He knew I wasn't coping too well. As for the hospital lifts I had cancelled them, as it was such a long wait to get a lift home as so many people had to rely on them. Thank God it worked out how it did.

Again I would never have left Mum to go on her own, but to say it was difficult was an understatement.

Mum coped amazingly well and the twenty-one days went surprisingly quickly.

After taking advice it was suggested that I should apply for Employment and support for Liam as it would mean more money, which they were desperate for. And it meant less trips into Newbury for him to sign on. At first he had to attend an appointment to be assessed. I told the lady doctor in the interview everything, about Liam, his problems as a child at school, then being statemented because of his problems with writing, reading and money, also reports from doctors confirming his difficulties. After asking many questions the only test she did was ask him to pick up a pencil, cup, and paper, then wave his hand in the order she requested of him for each task. What that proved I have no idea. Then spell word backwards which he couldn't do although he did think about it for a bit. I found all this very strange, well actually I found it stupid. What was she trying to find out from her daft little test? These wouldn't show how bad Liam was at reading, writing, or his lack of understanding money or his short term memory.

I hoped that the letters and doctors' reports were enough to prove that Liam had had these problems all his life. It was down in black and white written by consultants and doctors. (He would pass with flying colours surely?) I told her about the situation the children were left in, their mother dying and their father walking out on them. Everything I could think of she made notes on and then photocopied the lot, even the school reports requesting help for him during his lessons. And that he had been statemented, and allocated extra help during his lessons.

Two weeks later the report came back. He had scored zero in everything. The woman hadn't listened to anything or read anything, her test was crap and the reports and doctors' letters obviously counted for nothing. What an absolute waste of time. The reports weren't taken into consideration or his Dyspraxia; her test had not been suited to his problems and was utterly ridiculous for a boy with specific learning difficulties; in fact he had failed even before he had entered her office.

So that's when we got Orla a psychologist involved. (She was contacted for me through Connexions. They helped school leavers with jobs.) She came to the house and spent two long sessions with Liam testing his IQ, his spelling, his reading, maths, his memory, his common sense, working out puzzles, the meaning of words and phrases. It was the best thing we could have done as he was below average in most things, extremely low in others, one borderline and one average and that was only in his social skills. This was how the test should have been conducted. As soon as Employment and support received the new revised report they backtracked, and changed their decision. They also received a letter from Orla who I cannot thank enough. I have called on her a few times and each time she has helped. Liam isn't shirking work but there is so much he cannot do through no fault of his own and so few jobs for people like him with his type of disabilities. Whatever job he finds, it needs to pay more than his benefits as he is now the main bill payer. There is no Mum or Dad to cushion him and the little amount Lauren earns as an apprentice isn't enough. I give Liam an allowance each week, the rest is used for bills and shopping and any clothes needed. It is a difficult job to juggle everything, a complete worry and again my problem to make ends meet. But what happens when they have to move and there is rent to find? I know the money won't stretch that far. I cannot hand over the account for Liam to look after as God love him it would soon be drained, as he does not have the ability to run it himself.

My biggest worry is where they will eventually live when the house is sold? Diana had been too seriously ill to attend the court hearing a year earlier so a representative stood in for her. It didn't go as I had hoped or even thought it would. Sean was given £20,000 out of the mortgage money to pay off his debts. (He got married at a hotel, which wouldn't have been cheap, his choice! But what about his kids and their debts?) He was also rewarded seventy-five percent of the house after it is sold, the two kids will be left with just twenty-five percent. I have to find them somewhere to live; a boy on benefits and a girl on an apprentice hairdresser wage. The house is in very bad repair and will need much spending on it. I had part of the roof in the computer room mended (due to leaks) that cost £600+. I wish I hadn't paid for it now and just got it covered with a tarpaulin. Their account couldn't really afford being drained by that much. I could kick myself as they both need so much themselves but the ceiling would have probably come down so I had no choice but to pay a builder out of Liam's benefits.

Sean even had the cheek to request entry to the house to do it up and then the two kids pay half. That was the unbelievable bit! The solicitor rang him on their behalf as they didn't want him in the house, and no way were they paying anything. The solicitor's secretary told me that a lot of shouting went on mainly from him. I could quite believe it, as if Sean thinks he's right, then nobody else has an opinion. Later on there were other roof leaks, which my son covered with tarpaulin. The house can rot for all I care, it is nothing but a money pit. The wiring we have found out needs re-doing and a lot of old jobs from the past were badly done. If they were my kids whether they spoke to me or not would be my main priority. They would have half of the money no question about that; it would give them a better chance. Because of everything that has taken place they won't speak to him or see him and they absolutely loathe his new much younger wife.

It would be good if they could live in something smaller with maybe a little garden with maybe a garage. It would be perfect, nothing too old and not falling to pieces like their home is now, but somehow I don't think that is what they will get. I know I will have to take advice again as to how I proceed when the house is on the market. Newbury is a no no as they want to be near us all.

It will be another worrying time as I don't know how it will all turn out for them.

So much has happened and continues to do so; they deserve to be settled with no money worries and most of all happy and settled in their lives.

Chapter 26

In October – eight months after Diana's death, James became very ill. He and his girlfriend had split up a few months earlier; the reason is personal to them. I think that, and Diana's death caused him so much stress, and he had also decided to change jobs which as I said with hindsight wasn't the best decision. He was thrown straight in the deep end, he was expected to cold call businesses and try to sell industrial printers, having been told at the interview he would have training. Having had no experience of selling or even knowing enough about the product (only the books he was given to read) this put tremendous pressure on James. Now if it had been John or Mark they could sell ice to the Eskimos and coal to coalmen!

He was using the loo about twelve to fifteen times a day, bleeding, suffering pain, and bloating.

After many doctors' visits, he was then referred to the hospital. After seeing a specialist he told us that it sounded like he had all the symptoms of colitis. He was then immediately booked in for a colonoscopy, and on that same day he was diagnosed with ulcerated colitis. (Big shock even though we were told that's what it probably was.) James already suffered with IBS from a young age (about fourteen), I already had to watch his diet although some days he can eat anything then he'd have a flare up and it was back to bland non fibre food. He was started on steroids immediately and anti-inflammatories, he was also given an appointment to see the bowel consultant a few weeks later to see how he was managing on the steroids. These took a while to work as one particular area in his colon was still inflamed which was still bleeding and causing him discomfort. So it was decided by his consultant to admit James into hospital so they could get the disease under control as soon as possible (he was still using the loo about ten to twelve times a day and suffering tummy pain).

He was given a poo chart to fill in:

a) how many times he was going
b) what time?
c) what was the consistency?

(He said it was the most exciting time of his stay in hospital. Filling in the old poo chart was the highlight of his day, boredom sets in pretty quick!)

It took about three days before his bowel began to slow down, his pain became less and he looked better in himself. Luckily they had given him a room with his own loo as the urgency to go made it a rush to get to the loo. At one point he was asked to give up his room to someone else, he stuck up for himself saying that unless they wanted a mess every day in the corridors they had better let him stay put until he had improved and things had slowed down, (good for him I thought). He had one further stay in hospital just before Christmas as he was still experiencing problems and he was also finding it difficult to cope with the disease, it had completely taken over his life. He couldn't work or play his beloved football, or go out with friends as he had to be near a loo. He took to not eating if he was going out as he worried about his urgency and not making it to the loo. This I really worried about as not eating made him weak and tired, he was also becoming irritable and depressed.

His whole life was on hold as he waited for the medication to start working. Every time his steroids were reduced the condition flared up again. Now and again he met friends at the local pub but because he didn't eat before he went out he then got drunk very quickly. It then became difficult to persuade him to come home as it was obvious to me and Adam he was drowning his sorrows. (He says not but I'm sure being drunk made him forget about his illness.) The next day he couldn't even remember how he had made it home, I assumed a taxi, he didn't remember.

It was then that I would moan at him about spending money he couldn't afford and stupidly getting drunk while taking medication. Deep down I knew he needed to get out, it was difficult to know how to handle this as being in with me every day then on his own when I went out must have been driving him insane, as the world carried on without him. But the outings with mates only used up precious money.

After quite a few visits to see his consultant to tweak his medication and then introduce a new one, an immune suppressant, James has bad days and good days and has not yet been on the new medication long enough to see a drastic change. He has been assured that there are other things they can try, coming off the steroids will be the telling time. He cannot stay on them too long because of side effects. He takes calcium tablets to protect his bones, but only recently he fell and fractured the long bone in his arm, so he is now in plaster. No surprise there then!

He has regular blood tests and regular check-ups, no two days are the same for him. His diet is extremely bland and if he is tempted with something that upsets his tummy he suffers for a few days. If there was a way I would gladly let him have my colon (I'm fifty-three and done a bit and he is twenty-two and has so much in life to experience). Living with this disease is very unpredictable – a good day and you feel elated, a bad one you're looking for what may have upset his tummy. He's a lad after all, and lads are always hungry, they graze all day! It's times like these that I wish we humans just took tablets for food, daft I know but I hate seeing him like this. Being his mum I'd do anything to help my child no matter how old.

He recently saw a dietician and although we have been many times before, there are a few diet changes for him to try to help his condition.

He is now to drink Yakult every day and eat smaller portions, eat slower, and add ground linseed to cereals. He is not to reheat starchy food and so on and so on. I do hope these bloody well work because the cost is phenomenal and the disappointment is worse!

At present he is unable to work, as mornings are his worse; it takes a few hours for the steroids effects to kick in. Previous to his illness James had booked to do a personnel trainer course but he has had to put it on hold until things settle down.

He has had to sign on for a while and is now looking for a part-time job, hopefully afternoons (because of his difficult mornings). The money for S.S.P is minimal and not easy to budget as he still needs a car to get to and from hospital etc., so his father and I chip in with the cash when we can.

James can be very down some days as the illness takes its toll, it is very unpredictable and saps his energy. Making plans ahead often get altered because a good day can then become a bad day, hence the days he would get drunk to drown his sorrows. The less stress he has the better but it is a vicious circle.

I buy lottery tickets hoping that I can be the big winner (I dream about it all the time but unfortunately that's all it is) and sort out everyone's financial problems. Also Liam and Lauren's search for a home when the time comes and for James not to have money worries while he has ill health. This adds to his unneeded stress levels. Not good!

Life can be a real bitch as I have discovered these last three years.

We decided to spend Christmas with Liam and Lauren, in memory of Diana and her most favourite time of year; also it would be the last time they would spend Christmas here in their home. It was a bit of a squeeze in the little dining room. (John announced we should have set the table up in the sitting room because it was bigger.) Lunch was definitely noisy and not subdued as last year had been.

The best bit of course, the games at the end of the day as always! A couple of the boys' friends also turned up to join in with the games, news is getting around fast! And the competition between John, Mark and James grows every year, to be the big winner. I think next year to give the others a chance I will award the top prize to whoever comes last (won't say until all games are played). It was fun and noisy and not sad as the year before.

Kylie was heavily pregnant but still managed to look petite and she had a lovely glow about her.

Boxing Day was open house if anyone was at a loose end they could come to me for tea, which Liam and Lauren did and also Mum. James was also home for a while then went to watch the Boxing Day footy at the pub with his mates. John and Mark went to visit their dad in Weymouth.

I never like the months following Christmas. They are cold and damp with nothing to look forward to, only the warmer weather but that wouldn't be here for a long time, so January is always a bit of a nothing month, an anti-climax. Weight to lose, (AGAIN!) money to find as the bills for presents start to arrive. Empty bank accounts and empty food cupboards to restock. Cold after cold as the weather fluctuates from freezing to mild sometimes in one week, confusing the bulbs, confusing the birds and annoying the hell out of me.

This year we had another grandchild to look forward to, so it wasn't so bad this time.

Adam hates the winter months. He once stated that he suffers with S.A.D. in the winter. I just think he's cold all the time since his heart attack and thinks he suffers with it. I don't mind the darker evenings but I hate not seeing the sun shine, the dull cloudy days are depressing. Ah it's me that suffers with S.A.D!!!! Not him.

Rianne being born October 2009 was our first happy event then my second grandchild Olly was born on 18th February 2011. He is a gorgeous wonderfully natured little boy. I was told by phone that when he first opened his eyes Kylie thought he was the spitting image of me. 'He looks just like his nanny Jan,' she told me over the phone. I couldn't wait to see my little clone. When I did see him he had big eyes which have now turned dark brown like his father and me and looks so very like his father at the same age.

March arrived: we got through the anniversary of Diana's death pretty well. I invited everyone round for a special tea, the anniversary the 6th fell on a Sunday, which made it easier to be together. I couldn't quite believe a year had already gone, it only seemed like yesterday we had attended the funeral!

No matter how hard my mother must find it after losing a daughter, she hides her grief and keeps going for the sake of Liam and Lauren. There is never a day goes by when I don't think about my sister and I know my parents must be the same. To have a child die before you must be the worst possible tragedy ever. Nine or forty-nine they are still the child you bore and loved and then lost too early.

Our friend Mary had received bad news after finding a breast lump, she is presently undergoing chemotherapy and is being extremely brave. I wish her all the luck in the world and thank her for being a good friend to Diana and myself for a number of years.

After a few discussions and going through the pros and cons we decided to book a family holiday; eleven adults and two children. My father absolutely loves the seaside (who doesn't) and likes to be as near to the sea as possible, in it if he could! So I had to spend ages searching the Internet looking for the right property that had enough bedrooms, and loos, and near the sea and not too expensive. Not asking much then! It wasn't very easy. I also had to consider the travelling distance as neither of my parents wanted a long journey – so West Sussex was the best bet (they like that area) if I could find anything that is.

I had nearly given up when I found a beautiful large property right on the seafront, (The Breeze). Five bedrooms, four loos, two bathrooms, two showers and bags of space and the best bit: it was in West Sussex, West Wittering to be precise, even better. The price of £1200 per week split between us was very reasonable and only an hour and a half away from our homes. We were very lucky as it only had one week left in June. (One of the Wimbledon weeks but I'd get over it.) I booked it right away after informing everyone that it looked great and that if I didn't book it now we would lose it.

Agreed! Booked, done, yippee!

We now had a holiday to look forward to. Before that Mum still had a check-up due at the hospital. This we knew was due sometime in May; I just prayed that everything would be ok, as I didn't know what would happen if the cancer had returned. Or what the next step would be; this had not been discussed with us at the hospital. Also what about the holiday if things turned out bad? Luckily all was well; the check-up revealed no further cancer, the radiation had done its job.

I know Mum would have been reluctant for further radiation treatment, and we didn't even know if that would be an option for her. The treatment had worn her out and taken its toll on her wellbeing; to go through it all again at her age would be too much.

But thank you God (starting to believe again) all was well; I was so relieved for her. We left the hospital buzzing; a little bit of faith returned to me that day. I know as the weeks had been counting down Mum had been worrying about her six month check-up, now she could relax and look forward to a holiday.

The check-ups would continue regularly but for now luck was on our side, and boy didn't we deserve it.

Rita the wonderful neighbour opposite had agreed to look after Mable, Liam and Lauren's cat and keep an eye on the house.

James by now (just before the holiday) was dating a lovely girl called Louise, introduced to him by Liam (she is a friend of one of Liam's friends). He was animated when he came home after meeting her on their first date, not only did they like each other but she suffered with Coeliac disease (an intolerance to gluten) which had taken three years to diagnose so she understood exactly what James was going through when it came to urgent and frequent trips to the loo.

It too had taken over her life for a long time, as colitis was taking over James's although as long as Louise has a gluten free diet her condition is under control. I pray that James will soon have his condition under control, and he can eventually start his personnel trainer course, it is the right career for him and something he will enjoy doing.

Chapter 27

The Holiday

Friday 24th June 2011 we all set off for West Wittering in Sussex. The day was slightly cloudy but I was glad to see the sun shine. I took a couple of photos of Mum and Dad waving next to the car as we were about to set off.

'A very promising start,' my dad announced (referring to the weather) as he took his seat in the front of the car, (me and mum in the back).

It was a good journey and it didn't take long to reach the house which was fantastically huge (well in comparison to my home). The Breeze was exactly the right name for the house. When the back and front doors were open the sea breeze whipped through the house blowing everything that moved, hence each door had a secure hook attached to each wall otherwise everything would slam shut. There was never any chance of being too hot in the breeze, making me think of humid, uncomfortable summer days here in Berkshire; when it is hot it is impossible to keep cool. Those were the days when one would have loved to be sat in the breeze!

It was idyllic and completely safe and secure for Rianne who loved pushing her doll and pushchair from room to room in a circle. Kitchen to hall to dining room back to kitchen round and round she went, giggling all the time at her unexpected freedom. Chloe had also taken stair gates for extra safety. She was then free to roam. The garden was also fenced in, with a patio area and then a neat lawn, a path led to a gate then across to another gate, which led to The Breezes own private bit of the beach. How I envied the owners and the people that lived here along West Drive. Some of the houses were shut up which I felt sad about. If I owned a place like this I would be here every weekend.

Enjoying all it had to offer, for me the space, the peace, the view and the wonderful cooling salty breeze. Leaving all the problems behind for a whole week.

Not Cornwall, but the seaside all the same and an easier distance to do weekend trips.

The weather was kind to us, only the Saturday was cloudy so we decided to visit the sea life centre in Portsmouth. It was great fun and Rianne and Olly loved looking at the different fish; they had sharks, piranha, jellyfish, huge manta ray and a few creepy crawlies to look at. It certainly makes it more fun when you have children with you, they're excitement is infectious, which I must admit rubbed off on me.

We had lunch at a little café further along the seafront then finished the day in the arcades.

A very enjoyable fun day!

The rest of the week was hot so we had a bar-b-cue one day, drinking ice-cold lagers, heaven! Lazing around, watching Rianne paddling in the sea.

I wasn't so lucky during the bar-b-cue; I bit into a bread roll and broke a tooth in half. 'Bloody great,' it was a Sunday; so nothing would be open. I couldn't eat because the half that was left kept hitting the bottom tooth and bending, which bloody hurt.

So off I went with Adam to find a hospital to get some help. Although John had suggested he pull it out with the pliers he found in the garage. He had even sterilised them with Rianne's sterilizer tablets. You should have seen the dirty things that he presented me with assuring me that they were now clean and that one quick pull and he would have the tooth out. I won't repeat what I said to him.

It was so annoying to leave the bar-b-cue on the most perfect of days to look for the local hospital situated in Chichester about eight miles away. And I had been enjoying my lovely burger and creamy coleslaw. Sod's law. I am just drawn to hospitals, or they are drawn to me.

No luck when we got there. I was told emergency dental had already closed and that I should phone at five the next evening to make an appointment, but only if they could fit me in. It was getting better by the minute and my bloody broken tooth was really annoying me.

On the way back to The Breeze we called into a local shop to buy a few tins of soup as I knew I wasn't going to be able to eat the next day just slurp on liquid. Great!

Luckily John is persistent and as soon as morning arrived he was straight on the phone to National Health Direct to find me a dentist sooner rather than later.

At 12.10 Adam and I arrived in Portsmouth. John's persistence had paid off; I had to register as a new patient at a relatively new dentist in Portsmouth about fifteen miles from where we were staying. They would then see me. We only waited about half hour then I was called in. It was obvious to me that it was a very new practice as everything still had its shiny newness. The waiting room chairs looked hardly sat on and the walls were fresh and no marks were evident on any wall. The dentist numbed my mouth then pulled out the wobbly bit of my tooth, announcing she was unable to pull the root and that I would need to go to hospital if I wanted it out.

I knew my own dentist was capable of pulling out my root as she had already pulled out a couple of annoying and painful teeth for me. I had been petrified as I knew that one particular tooth had no more life in it and could not be filled anymore. This I had already been told by several other dentists. My options: have it removed at the hospital or let Abi (my dentist) pull it. She assured me that it would take her a matter of seconds to extract the large molar. She was as good as her word, the extraction did literally take seconds, twenty in fact! I counted. I didn't feel a thing. I hope she never leaves the practice, as I want no one else ever to pull my teeth. I hope I won't need any more pulled but you never know.

My tooth felt comfortable, although food kept getting trapped in the hole that had been left. So at bedtime I not only had to floss but stick the bristles of my toothbrush in and dig out any trapped food. I didn't want toothache the rest of the week. Life was never straightforward with me; I had decided that a long time ago. I wonder what life would have been like if I had been born a Leo and not a Gemini?

The rest of the week was warm, definitely beach and deckchair weather. We went to a few restaurants to eat and I made risotto a couple of times and Mum cooked as well. The kids behaved well and all in all we enjoyed the break. Unfortunately there had been a case of the Nora virus in the next village and guess what? Some of us got it. One by one we had bouts of sickness and diarrhoea, even the two children had bad tummies. Only three adults escaped it, I unfortunately wasn't one of them. Again it didn't surprise me; break a tooth, get a bug, easy peasy after the last three years! Still managed to enjoy the holiday though.

Chapter 28

My three sons are my pride and joy. I loved them as soon as they were first put into my arms and I love them just as much now.

John, the non-stop talker with his mobile phone glued to his ear nearly twenty-four-seven, who wants everything done yesterday like me. Short on patience but caring, a constant worrier, a joker and a quick wit. A great lover of football. He never stops running and works hard on the pitch. He plays every Sunday morning.

It took him forever when he left school to decide what he wanted to do. He had job after job moving from one to the next thinking it would be the one! But it never was as his boredom would set in and off he went again in search of the one that would bring a fortune. Thankfully and finally he chose bricklaying and has stuck at it and is very good at it. He leaves mess in his wake and is the untidiest person I know.

He wanted a son first and got a girl. She is the apple of his eye as I knew she would be.

His great love: Football. He watches, eats, breathes, and worships football. He probably talks about it in his sleep. Anything he can't find he blames Chloe for moving and storms around until it is found then apologises later for his tantrum.

Mark my middle son was the easiest, most contented baby in the whole world. He slept for England and still does. As a boy he was calm and not impatient like his older brother, he didn't chatter on like John preferring to be quieter. The complete opposite to his older brother, he is very tidy and organised. Unlike John he knew exactly what he wanted to do when he left school. He is a very talented joiner and has made many exceptional pieces of furniture. He also has a talent for making people laugh. He is an extremely good footballer and has played at a high standard! His name was taken by an Oxford United scout once at a tournament. If I had known more then I would have pushed for him to have a trial but his manager never mentioned it again and it was forgotten about. He was always organised and tidy at home. He got his homework done then went out with his friends while John spent the whole evening moaning about doing it and didn't have as long out, because of the moaning and the amount of time it took to do his homework. I told him once that if he did it without a fuss he would be out the same time as Mark, it didn't work. John, listen? That's a laugh!

James my youngest was another easy baby; incredibly funny as a toddler, full of chatter and confidence. An incredible footballer from the day he struck a ball and at seven he was picked up by Chelsea Football Club and taken on their books at eight. He was there until he was thirteen and then he moved on to Southampton F.C. At fourteen he was diagnosed with irritable bowel and it has been that and now colitis that has stopped him from reaching the top in the sport. John his brother has said all along that somebody up there never wanted him to be a professional footballer. I must say I believe him now. Something always happened that got in his way: he broke his growth plate in his ankle at eleven, it took him ages to get his form back, and his confidence, then he got glandular fever at fifteen and again missed nearly a season of football, then he went down with a bad case of chicken pox. His IBS would flare up at the wrong time and now colitis has been the final straw. He can't imagine not playing some kind of football. I pray he gets better soon and his life can be normal once again.

The three girls in my sons' lives are all great; Chloe is daft, soft, incredibly kind, and funny without even realising it, she puts people's feelings first and worries about them. She is easy to talk to and phones me every day to check how everything is going. She is a great mum to Rianne. She is the right girl for John as you need the patience of a saint to cope with his chatter (his phone is constantly stuck to his ear) and the stress moods he gets himself into. They both live in complete chaos and are well suited.

Kylie we didn't meet for nearly six months because of her shyness. We would hear them come in then a little squeak from the hall which I believed to be a hello then she'd run upstairs with Mark. Some days she even got as far as waving from the hall doorway; we never quite saw her face.

She is absolutely fine now her shyness gone, she is a real character with her animated chatter, funny expressions and girlie ways. She calls Olly 'her olly dolly' and is so pleased to at last have a baby. She is dinky in size. She probably pouts at Mark and gets her own way, although it could be the other way round as I think she would do anything for Mark. They are opposite to John and Chloe: very tidy and organised.

Louise has just entered the family and is James' girlfriend. Straight away she has slotted right in, she chats easily and we all liked her from the start. She understands about James' illness and what he is going through as she herself suffers with coeliac disease and had three very difficult years herself before the condition was diagnosed. Which makes it less embarrassing for him, because she understands so well the problems he goes through every day. She giggles at him when he makes her laugh. Already she has been to the pictures with Lauren and Chloe and they have shopped till they dropped. She has taken Lauren for lunch. Lauren likes her very much. She has confidence and is friendly.

She is dinky as well, the job she does is a difficult one (she works with autistic children/teenagers) and has been hit several times, but she sticks at it and enjoys her work.

As long as they all love each other and look after each other I couldn't ask for more.

Chapter 29

James's colitis took a turn for the worse. His steroids didn't kick in until the afternoons which meant he couldn't be away from a toilet in the mornings, and as soon as the steroids were reduced his bowel became even more inflamed. In a whole year he has not been able to come off them. He was started on immune suppressants and told it would be a few weeks before they began to work, all we could do was hope that they did.

On 14th August 2011 Rianne and Olly were christened. It was more like a wedding reception as so many family and friends were there. The church was packed. It was a perfect day; the weather was brilliant, bright and sunny. And the two children were great when it came to the wetting of heads at the font with the lady vicar. Not a peep from either of them, except the chatter from Rianne, which had me giggling in my seat. The service was a bit long, (well longer than when mine were christened) but it was lovely and very special. I was knackered from all the food preparation but then so probably were Chloe, Kylie, their mums and sisters. Even my dear mum and Lauren helped out as they worked very hard to make sure there was enough to feed everyone. Need not have worried there was more than enough with plenty left over!

Rianne wore a white dress with a pink trim and pink shoes and a white headband. Olly wore a white trouser suit with a pale blue waistcoat. What a picture they both were. Gorgeous! My special wonderful grandchildren!

James nearly didn't make it as again he was having a bad day, but at the last minute turned up and stood at the back of the church in case he needed to dash to the loo.

These are the times I miss Diana more than any other time, knowing she would have enjoyed the christening and helping out with the food. It is sad that she isn't here to enjoy occasions like these. She would have adored my two (now three) grandchildren as she did her nephews. I know she would have been with us in spirit watching the special day and happy that Liam and Lauren were asked by Chloe and John to be Rianne's Godparents.

Mum has told me since that she had been dreading the day, as she hadn't been in a church since Diana's death. But as always she coped and was entertained by the sheer excitement and noise of it all.

The following week Adam and I left for a holiday in Cornwall, this time we stayed on a farm, in a converted barn. We were away from the farmhouse; in front of us fields and the sea. In the fields were various animals, sheep, cows, and a couple of goats. And apart from the obvious animal noises, complete and utter peace.

We were near St. Just, in the district of Pendeen not far from Lands End. We could travel every day and not meet a car for ages. I wondered if the people that lived here realised just how lucky they were, such peace and beauty, so different to where we lived. I'm sure they must, how could you not?

The farm owners had only been in Cornwall for fifteen years, they had moved from Lancashire because they too fell in love with the beauty and tranquillity of Cornwall.

This holiday was just sheer utter lolling and laziness; we relaxed and enjoyed every minute of our visit. We visited many places that we hadn't been to before ambling around the different quirky villages, visiting book shops as we both love books. Mostly we stayed outdoors because the weather was fantastic, stopping at little seaside cafés, marvelling in the scenery whilst drinking cold, ice filled drinks. Stopping for lunch where we wanted then moving on to sit by the sea book in hand with a view to die for. The weather was extremely hot so it definitely wasn't a holiday for rushing about. Thank heavens for the air con in the car to cool us once hot from our mooching around the various hamlets.

We love the Lizard and Tintagel, and try to go to as many places as possible to wander around the narrow streets taking in the loveliness of it all. The busier places like Polperro and Perronporth and the quiet charm and quaintness of Mousehole, and the amazing Minnack Theatre; a work of art and a project of incredible dedication. All of these places I would go back to time and time again and never tire of them.

After having three kids I always needed to find a loo wherever we went. I did do my pelvic floor exercises after each child but it never made any difference, it became a joke between us that it wasn't park and ride but park and pee.

Luckily there are many public loos about so I never had to worry and I always carry my own supply of loo roll just in case!

By the end of the week we were bronzed, relaxed, and pounds heavier. Well I was. Adam still does his cardiac exercises even on holiday. I did join in for two nights but got bored and sat eating chocolate raisins while I watched him. Hard work, chewing!

My will power left me three years ago, and my got up and go, got up and went long before that. I hope to get it back when I have finally found Liam and Lauren a home and all the Ts are crossed and the Is are dotted so to speak. Think I heard that in A Christmas Carol used by Scrooge. I liked it.

So with tighter fitting clothes we headed home. As it was raining for the first time that week it wasn't such a wrench to leave our favourite place; I know we will be back next year. I'm thinking of writing another book called Park and Pee for all the ladies with my problem. Detailing the best loos to use as I think I have visited nearly all the loos in Cornwall!!

Chapter 30

It was decided when we got home because time was moving on we should think about packing up things and getting rid of rubbish at the house. I didn't want everything left until the last minute as there was a lot of stuff to sort out that had been collected over the years. Lauren turned eighteen in October, the house then had to be sold.

Being such a big job it was out of the question to keep making trips to the dump so the best idea was hiring a skip and getting rid all in one go. So Adam took a day off and with Liam, Lauren, myself, Mum and their friend Mike, we began sorting through and then turning out the unwanted rubbish. Unbeknown to us Sean had been watching the house. He called the police and said we were having a garage sale with his belongings; he evidently had seen a van taking away some furniture from the next door neighbours and assumed we were selling stuff.

Even if we had decided to sell stuff which I might add we hadn't, it was legal, as he had missed the deadline to claim any rights to any items in the house, these now belonged to the two children. We showed the police the rubbish in the skip and said Sean was welcome to any of it because it was rubbish. I offered the policeman a rusty old kettle, funnily enough he declined.

From the window we could see Sean grumbling away to the police at the top of the road, but they asked him to leave, as we were not breaking any laws. Whatever we had done over the last few years he always saw the bad in it. He would turn up at my home moaning and groaning about the mortgage or blaming me for the kids not wanting to see him, which hand on heart is completely untrue. I remember once when things were incredibly difficult with Diana and tensions were high and arguments were many, I had to shout Lauren down during one particularly difficult day because we couldn't do anything to change what was happening. She became very upset, I asked her if she wanted to see her father, maybe that would help, but she got cross and said he was the last person she wanted to see.

The only thoughts in Liam and Lauren's heads now was their mother and how much they missed her. When she was seriously ill they never once mentioned their father. No one can imagine how hard it was for them to watch her slowly and painfully deteriorate each day.

Once we had completely filled the skip it felt very good, the garage looked neat and tidy, as it looked like an explosion before we started. We were filthy, tired but very satisfied with our very hard work. Mike had helped Liam empty the loft, another big job completed. Liam works very hard once you gee him along.

We spent the next few weeks packing boxes and taking old clothes to the charity collection sites.

I remember we all coughed a lot because of all the dusty items we were handling.

Some of the packing up boxes were taken over to Rita's to store as wherever they moved to it would be smaller than this home. They couldn't take everything but some things had sentimental value and had belonged to Diana.

The biggest job had been the garage and the loft, we could now store some of the packed boxes in the empty garage; these were the things that would go with Liam and Lauren. At last the house was looking emptier, we couldn't do anything about the flat roof or the saliva stained carpets as there wasn't enough money to put these things right. Whoever bought it would have to spend a fortune, the best bet would be builders buying it then gutting it and starting again. The garden had defeated us a long time ago, Liam would cut the grass but nobody went near it when Diana was alive, there wasn't time and it wasn't important, she was.

I knew it would sell though because of its position; a quiet no through road, a large garden, room to park two or three cars, room to extend and very near the primary and secondary schools and local shops. It was once a lovely family home, it would be again. The memories would go with us!

Chapter 31

James had another appointment at the hospital. His immune suppressants had not made any difference, and there was nothing else to try. His only other choice was to have his colon removed, have a bag and then later on have reconstruction. James took it better than I thought he would. In fact so did I, as his life at the moment was non-existent; no job, no sport, no money and a very embarrassing illness to cope with. If a year ago it had been the only option, we would have left with very heavy hearts, but now a year on it was controlling every aspect of his life. Removing the colon got rid of the disease and gave him back his life; we left feeling a bit subdued but positive. It wouldn't have been his choice but it was his only choice so accept it he did. As he said when we got back to the car just to go walking again and not worry where the loo was or get up and eat breakfast and not starve himself and to play football again, it would all be worth it.

I was very proud at the way he handled the news from his doctor. John would have never accepted it, he told me that himself. I'm not so sure as you have to experience something to know how you would really feel.

His operation would be in about two months' time, giving him a bit of time to come to terms with it all.

He had been given plenty of booklets to read, step by step on the operation, the stoma itself, feelings after such a big operation, reconstruction. James read it all, any information he couldn't get he would look it up on the Internet. Also people's experiences, which were quite varied.

John's thirtieth birthday on September 8th was celebrated at our local football club, with a very good D.J., cooking done by yours truly, also Kylie, Chloe and Chloe's mum. Very knackering but the evening was good fun. Rianne ran around the hall loving every moment and olly slept surprisingly through the loud music in his pushchair. Worst bit was clearing up at the end, so we couldn't leave until the place was cleared and left as we found it.

For James's and Lauren's birthdays we decided to book a table at a popular eating place near Reading, The Mansion House. About ten miles from us, it was a joint celebration of Lauren's eighteenth and James's twenty-second. The grandchildren sitting in highchairs as good as gold, both chatting away, Olly with his baby chat and Rianne, her speech getting better by the day amusing us all.

Then on the following Tuesday – Lauren's actual birthday we all met up as usual for tea and cake and chat. Lauren also had many outings to go to at the weekend with friends and colleagues – after all you're not eighteen everyday!

It was so difficult for Liam and Lauren celebrating birthdays and Christmas and not having Diana here to celebrate with them.

At the tea party was James, Liam, Mary, my mum, Chloe and Rianne. The room was pretty crowded, Mum had made a birthday cake and we all sang Lauren happy birthday. We didn't know it then but their father was just about to force them out of their home.

It was late afternoon; Mum had been in the back garden picking up eating apples as she often did so she could make them and my dad apple crumble with thick custard. Just previously a white van had sped past the house then turned round and took off at a great speed, why it didn't ring alarm bells I don't know.

Mum had just come back in from the garden when I think it was Chloe shouting that Sean was in the back garden. He had come over the back fence, as I got to the kitchen there he was with some dopey looking boy who was filming with I think his mobile phone. 'I'm taking back the house,' he said as he locked the back door behind him. He isn't a pleasant guy when confronted and he had a menacing look on his face which is very scary at times.

I immediately phoned the police while Lauren stood shouting at her father to leave; he had chosen to come on her eighteenth birthday, what kind of person does that? We were all in total disbelief, the whole time the dopey looking boy kept filming. I tried to phone the solicitors but he had obviously waited until the offices were closed until he got in.

By then my other sons had turned up. John the oldest told him to go and how could he do it to his own kids? His reply, 'They made me suffer for four years now it was their turn.'

This I was told later – his life had been hell? What about them losing their mother. Wasn't that the biggest hell anyone could go through? This bloke had no compassion and was a complete and utter fool. He was the kid. My niece and nephew have more about them than he ever will!

My mum had gone to pieces, she needed to get home it was too much for her. Her health was delicate and she was too old to cope with the angry exchanges. Chloe also left and took Rianne to the top of the road as the shouting was frightening her.

By now some woman was trying to get into the house, Sean darted forward to open the door. John pushed him out so that he could lock the door but Sean grabbed him around the neck and pulled John out towards him, James went to help and the three of them fell through the fence, which is covered in a plant with sharp prickles.

I dropped the phone and ran outside as I could see Sean's wife grabbing at James. I grabbed at her cardigan which slipped through my fingers and she grabbed towards me calling me a bitch. Takes one to know one!

I can't begin to tell you how many police cars arrived as neighbours had also called the police. I'd say at least six.

It was more like Gangs of New York than a peaceful little known road.

The police asked us to return into the house, so we could explain what was going on. I thrust the court order under one policeman's nose, who informed me they didn't deal with domestics and it really was a solicitor's job.

I explained that it was Lauren's eighteenth and that it had been their home with their mother until she died and that he had left and hadn't lived there for four years. Also the house was on the market and when sold I would need to find his children a home.

His story – he told the police that him and his wife had been attacked – now why didn't we think of that? He had got my son by the throat but I was more concerned at keeping him out and the children in the only home they had ever known.

It became obvious to me that he had already planned this – get us arrested, he gets back into the house which he hadn't paid towards anything for two years, it had to be sold anyway why not leave them in peace for a few more weeks?

And that is just what happened, me, a fifty-three-year-old menopausal women got read my rights along with John and James for supposedly attacking him and his wife. We were led from the house, he stood across the road with a smirk on his face, which funnily enough didn't bother me as I hadn't attacked anyone, and I had done nothing wrong. The truth is stronger than a lie, liars have very short memories.

We had been through far worse than this losing my sister. I knew we would be ok. It was always Liam and Lauren that suffered in the end. Behind me I left them distraught and inconsolable. Liam was pale and in shock. Don't ask me what makes a man turn against his own children. Isn't it a parent's job to nurture, forgive, understand? Obviously not their father. I can understand now why they want nothing to do with him.

Back to the police station! I was DNA'd, photographed, searched and finger printed and then for five and a half hours the three of us sat in separate cells waiting to be interviewed. The cell was empty apart from a toilet and a sink built into the wall, and a mattress; that was it, nothing to look at or do. Can't say it was a pleasant experience and I was worrying about back home and what was happening to my poor niece and nephew. Being arrested is also an extremely good laxative as the nerves took over and my colon went into overdrive. Sitting on the cell toilet pebble dashing it at least five times, then running out of the loo roll I had been given. (A small box containing about 20 sheets.) I had to ring for more which ended up being this hard blue stuff you see in garage forecourts. Bloody marvellous, they had run out just when I was in colon cleanse! There I sat on the bog with a camera trained on me, my large white control pants around my ankles not caring who was watching, although I have since been told that the loo part is blacked out for privacy. But I don't know how true that is.

I had a long time to sit and reflect as to how we ended up in this situation. And I felt so angry that James had been arrested. He had enough to cope with, the colitis sapped all his strength, my only relief was that he too had a loo if his colitis should flare up.

While we were locked in our cells, Rita who had arrived back home to help the distraught kids, witnessed from her window Sean's wife making scratches on his back. Louise and Chloe also saw this happen, and immediately told the police what they had just witnessed. This was obviously to make it look like Sean had been badly hurt.

My only thoughts were where were the two children? I was told in my interview that they had been allowed fifteen minutes to grab as much as they needed for that night then they could come back later on to get the rest of their stuff. I sat there crying as the policeman in my interview told me that Lauren, in front of neighbours, Sean, and his wife carried out her mother's ashes sobbing her eyes out. He did not bat an eyelid one word comes to mind and that is heartless!

I was shown a photograph they had taken of his wife, she had her arm held out which showed a long deep gash on it which I had supposedly inflicted on her. It was utterly pathetic as I had not touched her skin, she had also been wearing a brown cardigan – which she was not wearing in the photo and the other thing she obviously didn't know about is I bite my nails so what was I supposed to have scratched her **with**? The flick knife I carry or the bowie knife I keep tucked in my knickers???? Idiots!

I cried then as I hate liars and because it was so very traumatic and I was by now very tired. I felt like a criminal and helpless because I didn't know what was going on at home, and how upset those two children must be.

What upset me more than anything were the lies. I tell white lies, we all do, but these were great big whopping black ones aimed at getting me into serious trouble.

Once the police had the whole story it became obvious what they thought about the incident. John had hand marks and scratches on his neck. Guilty? Only of trying to look after Liam and Lauren and make sure they didn't lose their home, and enough money to live on and food on the table. Guilty? Of helping them get over the death of their mother, that's all!

We finally left the station at one-thirty a.m. and I cried again when I saw the boys and they were ok, then spotting Adam and Chloe getting out of our car. I just wanted a cup of tea and my bed and to know how my niece and nephew were.

Adam (he is such a great guy) took the next day off as he was tired, it had been a very long night! And there was so much to sort out. As soon as morning arrived I rang the solicitors. We could go in at ten to see our solicitor.

Liam and Lauren had spent the night on my mum's sofas. They didn't sleep much which was to be expected, they looked pale and pretty scared when we called in to see them. Lauren announced, 'We're homeless now, Aunty Jan. Dad must really hate us.' I hugged them both.

'I'll sort it,' I told them, 'just bear with me.' I laughed when she told me that she had brought all the telly controllers with her so no one in the house could operate the T.V.s. What a girl! All that upset and she remembers to grab the remotes.

The first place we went to was housing to see if they could help. We had quite a wait as the place was very busy; women with small children and various other people from all walks of life all waiting for the same as us, a home. All they could offer was a hostel in Newbury.

'I'm not putting my niece and nephew in a hostel, they don't deserve that,' I replied indignantly. We were just one of many waiting for some kind of help. No wonder the women who worked there looked stressed they just didn't have the accommodation to offer unless Lauren had three kids then something would have had to be found. I couldn't do the job these people did. Many homeless not enough homes, too many waiting on long lists. We were eventually taken to a room and any points they might have were worked out (the more points the more chance of bidding for a home). You need quite a few to qualify for some kind of housing, working it out I think they probably only qualified for a wheelie bin! Joking apart our only option; claim housing benefit and rent privately, because of Liam's disabilities and because he was on ES@A and DLA he stood a good chance of getting quite a bit of help. I just needed to do more phone calls and form filling and gather evidence of what he received and prove that as an apprentice Lauren only gets £2.50 an hour. I would need her wage slips and up to date statements. We felt a tiny bit more positive but it would take time and staying at my mum's wasn't fair to any of them. They had no beds to sleep on, we also had to find storage for the immense amount of stuff they had in the house. I had the feeling again of being overwhelmed as we left for the solicitors. For the last four years nothing had been straight forward, would it ever be again?

At the solicitors we sat around a large shiny table in what I supposed was a conference room.

The outlook wasn't too bad as it meant applying back to the court to enforce the court order. An order to sell the house would take a bit of time, Sean could stay there but it wouldn't be for long.

He, I was told had installed security cameras, God knows why. None of us wanted to go anywhere near that road or him, what a waste of money! The solicitor suggested the mortgage payments were stopped as the children were no longer living there. Too right, let him sort it out. I emailed her back agreeing to her suggestion.

What he had hoped to achieve I don't know; upset and hurt his kids? He'd done that. Make life difficult? Yeah he'd done that. But life had been difficult ever since he had left them, we were used to all of the above, coping with Diana had been far harder than anything that happened after that.

He left because he didn't love Diana anymore. Fair enough it happens all the time, but you can't leave and then try and dictate what happens after that. He walked away but expected his children to accept it and still see him, and accept his then girlfriend. They chose not to see him, or accept her, they were angry and hurt. Which is their right. They wanted to protect their mother and hated seeing her cry and struggle day to day, and it wasn't long before the illness started to rear its head.

She became their only priority not their father.

They were allowed back into the house a few days later, at first Sean said only Liam and Lauren were allowed in but the police pointed out to him that they couldn't carry out heavy furniture on their own so my son Mark and his friend Sam went in to help. Sean watched through the lounge window videoing everything that was taken; it belonged to the kids anyway so it made no difference. He had already bagged up a lot of stuff, in some black sacks. Him and his wife had thrown rubbish from the bins mostly on Lauren's clothes. This we knew was retaliation because when the kids had been forced to leave Lauren had emptied everything she could get her hands on onto the floor in the kitchen. She had, through her tears, upset and anger emptied the utensil drawers of their contents throwing them around the room, she had pulled down her curtains in her bedroom and left it in a mess. Although Lauren's room was always the typical teenage hovel, so it wasn't a lot different, at times she would get a burst of enthusiastic energy and completely blitz the place.

She had left it as messy as time allowed, she told me that the police who had escorted them in told her not to make a mess. Apparently she turned to the two police chaps and snapped, 'How would you feel if your father had forced you out of your home?' You've got to admire her! Well I do. The police said nothing more while she did her deeds.

Liam and Lauren have some really great friends and they rallied helping with as much as they could. Her friend Carly's parents offered their garage to store larger items, Sam offered his lock-up and Mum's small lounge became home to the smaller items. Rita already stored a bit and took even more; everything was found a home. It proved difficult to sort out the clothes they needed for day to day as there were many sacks to look through and Lauren needed to locate her college books which had been put somewhere, but where we didn't know. We had to sit on the floor and go through bag after bag until everything they needed was located. Things that were not so important I brought home and kept in my spare bedroom, at least we knew now where to lay our hands on things. It wasn't ideal living at my mum and dad's, they were used to peace and quiet. Liam and Lauren were typical youngsters, noisy and full of energy. I would get different versions from young and old of various events taking place; Mum's version, then Liam's and Lauren's. All I took with a pinch of salt as it wasn't fair to any of them to live like this, they deserved their own homes and to just be grandparents and grandchildren again.

They were uncomfortable on the blow-up beds. I had purchased a double for Liam and Carly, Lauren's friend lent her a blow-up bed she used for camping. Both kids longed for their own comfy beds and a home of their own.

Liam missed his computer, his X-box and his Sky music channels.

They spent a lot of time with me as they didn't have a room of their own to just chill away from everyone, my house is pretty full up but I let them watch the programmes they liked and they could help themselves to snacks and use the computer and Liam could play the X-box with James. When they went home Mum and Dad were usually in bed then they could watch a bit of telly and make some supper, which Mum didn't mind. Dad is a bit more set in his ways, with old fashioned values.

'Kids are to be seen and not heard.' I think they were a bit wary of my father so kept out of his way, only because he was glued to the telly, watching his beloved cricket which the kids would find as boring as hell. I felt equally sorry for them all so I needed to get something in place ASAP.

I spoke to many people in the next few weeks. The housing benefit claim form was sent for me to complete and I requested banks statements for Liam, I sorted out his letters to prove he received DLA and E&SA and got Lauren to find as many payslips as she could and a bank statement.

I had to try and find them somewhere to rent that was affordable. What I didn't bank on was that a lot of people (due to bad experiences) refuse to let to people on benefits, and even when I explained that Liam had learning difficulties and it wasn't that he didn't want to work it made no difference. Some of the rental companies said they would speak to the various landlords and explain the situation. Some just said no right off. There were only a few flats to go after but they were turned down each time. I don't think it was so much where the money was coming from but the fact that they were young and also brother and sister. A lot of landlords want professional people and assume all youngsters will be party animals, and not responsible enough to look after someone else's property. This unfortunately does happen as I have heard stories before of property being disrespected, giving all youngsters a bad name.

This was going to be harder than I thought, but I persevered and pestered and in some cases pleaded their case and at last found a sympathetic ear, I suggested they meet Liam and Lauren and see for themselves what nice kids they are and because I am Liam's appointee and took care of bills etc. on their behalf there would, I promised, never be a shortfall in rent or the bills.

And at long last I found the perfect flat for them and before Christmas – even better. I hoped now things were looking up and 2012 would be a change for the better. The first thing I went out and bought them was a Christmas tree and decorations for their new home. Now hopefully new beginnings!

Chapter 32

James received his appointment to have his operation, the date they wanted him in was 11th November, he would stay in between four to seven days depending how he was after the operation. I was relieved, it gave him enough time to recover fully before Christmas as he had a few things arranged. One was staying at my niece's house in Yeovil during Christmas week, the other was a show that Louise had arranged in London as part of his Christmas present. These he was eager to do.

While James had his stay in hospital it would coincide with Liam and Lauren's move to their new home. Once James had been in a couple of days the move would take place that following weekend. It wasn't ideal but it was just sod's law it worked out like that. At least James would be recovering and Louise had already arranged to be with him on the Saturday of the move, we would then visit the next day. This move would be hard as so much stuff was coming from so many places. The flat would probably burst at the seams because of the amount of their belongings. It would take many weekends and evenings to sort out, as things had to be looked through and sorted into keep, store, or get rid of. To be honest I was dreading it; my mind was purely on James and how he would be once he first set eyes on his stoma.

I have always been a worrier, I remember when I was a lot younger saying to my first husband that, 'I was worried.'

He asked what was worrying me.

I replied, 'I don't know, it's because I haven't got a worry that I'm worried.'

Nuts, yeah! I think what I meant was when I hadn't got something to focus on I got the feeling of dread that something was going to happen, but I didn't know what. Double nuts! Even I don't understand myself sometimes, must be a Gemini thing.

James was understandably nervous, on the other hand he wanted his life back, this disease dictated everything he could and couldn't do.

We were all relieved when it was time to leave for the hospital. It was very early, James had to be there by seven a.m. He was first on the list to be operated on, his op was due at nine a.m., still quite a wait. Even the nurse thought it was a bit early, as it wasn't only James that had to be at the hospital by seven; anyone else due for surgery that day had to be there by seven, so imagine how long they had to wait. His letter requested seven a.m. so seven a.m. we got him there for.

He was asked by the nurse on duty to change into a hospital gown. We had annoyingly forgotten his slippers so it was very funny when he appeared from the cubicle wearing a pea green gown, tight dark green socks to stop deep vein thrombosis and fluorescent green ballet style slip on shoe things. Everyone in the waiting room started to laugh as he looked like a ballet dancing runner bean. James joined in with the laughing as he knew how daft he looked and it broke the silence. I promised that we would return later with his slippers adding that I preferred the footwear he had on!

At nine on the dot he was collected. We walked with him as far as we were allowed, I hugged him, then we left. I felt tearful as I knew how nervous he was, the waiting is what makes it even harder for any patient.

We headed straight home to pick up his slippers, then returned straight away as I wanted to be near the hospital. We had breakfast at Morrisons, then did a bit of shopping. I had no idea how long the surgery would take, there was no point returning to the ward until after one p.m. as that would be the earliest we could see him. It was also pointless going home as it was quite a way to keep travelling back and forth and anyway I didn't want to go anywhere else. Mr Arnold the surgeon always rang waiting relatives once the patient was in recovery. I kept my phone on loud because I didn't want to miss his call, so until we received that phone call we had time to kill. We had lunch in the hospital canteen then later on we had a coffee at the Costa Coffee shop. By two we still hadn't heard anything which made me a bit panicky as he had gone at nine. How long was his bloody colon? I had visions of them pulling his long diseased colon for hours until the thing finally plopped out, yuk!

Adam as usual told me I worried too much, um, an understatement. The nurse on the front desk told us that he wasn't back yet after ringing down to check on his whereabouts; apparently the op hadn't started on time and to check with them again at four.

Finally at three-thirty my mobile rang and Mr Arnold said that James was fine, everything had gone well and that he was now in recovery and to make my way to the ward at about four-thirty.

My relief was immense, he was ok and I would see him soon.

As we approached his bed he looked pretty duffed up. He was wearing an oxygen mask and had tubes coming from various parts of his body. He lifted a weak hand when he saw us then promptly told me off as my mobile started to ring.

'Turn it off, Mum,' he snapped.

'Ok, James,' I replied as I clicked the offender off.

He was very groggy and slipped in and out of sleep. We sat there quietly, pleased to at last see him.

He occasionally opened his eyes to check we were there giving us a weak sleepy smile. Nurses came to his bed regularly to check his blood pressure and his pee bag, which he hadn't been too happy about but a necessity he had been told by the stoma nurse. It was there to drain excess fluid and of course his pee. He needed to stay in bed until the next day when he was then expected to have a gentle walk around the corridors. Things are so different now. When my mum had me and Diana, a new mum stayed in hospital for two weeks to recuperate.

Staying in or sat by your bed the whole time, now it's more like op, up and out! Any problems call your own doctor; as usual it's all about money and the number of beds needed.

James's second day was the first time he saw the stoma; this made him tearful as his stoma nurse had said it would. Also the anaesthetic can make a person's mood low. I remember this from my own op when I had half of my thyroid removed in my thirties. I spent one day crying for no apparent reason, I couldn't say what the problem was but I remember feeling very depressed and sat in my nightie all day bawling my eyes out not even stopping when the boys came in from school! The next day I felt completely fine just a bit sore but not too bad.

James rang me at home sounding very down asking me to come in as soon as I could get there. I knew he was tearful by his voice. I didn't argue, I just rang Adam, explained how James felt and waited for him to pick me up.

When I got to the ward my sister and brother-in-law had arrived from Dorset to visit him. I didn't mention his tearful phone call in front of them as he was doing his best to join in the conversation. He was still very sleepy so his talk was limited. He is very fond of his aunty and uncle so it actually cheered him up by the end of their visit.

Over the next few days his colour and his mood returned although he couldn't face food for a while. He managed to sip a drink and attempted to nibble the corner of a sandwich, but fancied nothing for the first few days.

He had a morphine drip attached to him and could administer this himself. By pressing a button he could allow a small amount into his arm, he couldn't overdose because it was set so it could only be used every five minutes a few drops at a time.

His insides must have been very bruised and painful; it was no surprise that food was the last thing he wanted. He was given nutritional drinks to aid his recovery.

I didn't see his stoma until he came home. He needed my help at first, cutting the stoma bag to the correct size and generally getting things ready like his wipes and waste bags and getting used to this alien thing. You can't control its contents; even while you change the bag the bloody thing leaks like a tap, so you have to cover it with the special gauze supplied to stem the flow while you clean and reapply the bag. It isn't the most attractive thing, it's like a huge blood red boil, but very neatly done by Mr Arnold and it would shrink in size over the coming weeks hence having to cut the stoma bag to fit over it. I was actually very impressed. It is part of him, it has given him back his life, and he has now accepted it and copes with it brilliantly. The nurse said to him before his op, don't worry about it, and live your life normally; he is doing just that.

His girlfriend isn't bothered by it she loves him unconditionally. He calls it 'his bag of shite.'

He now has to fully recover and decide whether he wants to have reconstruction and get rid of the stoma. The next stage is a very big op, it means creating a pouch inside the stomach made from his own small intestine, then the stoma is pushed back into the stomach. The tricky bit is retraining the new bowel to hold its contents. The patient still needs to go about four or five times a day minimum and always once at night, so it is a big decision for James to make. The pouch does eventually break down which means the patient will after about twenty-five years return to a colostomy bag, unless they come up with another option/improvement over the coming years. Hopefully this will be the case and he won't need a stoma ever again. In the meantime he can work again until he decides what he would like to do.

He has had a few check-ups and will continue to have these at regular intervals.

James is contacted once a month by Medilink to take his order on colostomy bags, gauze and wipes etc. This will continue as long as he has a stoma; the order is then delivered by Parcel Force straight to the door.

Any concerns he has he can phone the stoma nurse and request an appointment if needed. And be seen pretty quick.

He is already talking about holidays and trips out, things that were near on impossible before his op, and finding a good job, changing his car and going back to sport. It is so nice to hear, as before it was all about where the nearest loos were!

For whatever reason Sean decided not to stall on the sale of the house, probably seeing what needed doing to it and that he was getting quite a bit of money. He let the estate agents show round potential purchasers. It went under offer pretty quickly, just as the estate agent said it would. The asking price was offered and accepted by Sean and the two children had to give their agreement. There was no reason not to as they needed money behind them. We have been able to put some of the money away for when either of them marry, some for a car each when they pass their tests. Lauren bought a hamster and Liam an aquarium, also a few bits and pieces they needed for the flat.

They love it even though it is much smaller, they feel safe.

The employment and support stopped and the help from the council ceased. This will all continue again once the money has depleted to a certain amount. Liam will always receive Disability Living Allowance money as this is permanent.

They have adjusted quite well to living in a much smaller space, but they feel safer away from their old home and it is so much warmer than the drafty old place they were made to leave. They also argue quite a bit, but they make up very quickly.

I often wish things were different for them and that they had the close family they once had. I will never be their mother but I am always here and always will be.

Chapter 33

Update

This has been an extremely difficult book to write, but I needed to get it out of my head and heart and down on paper. It has helped me to come to terms with what happened to my dear sister. Although I can't accept it because she had so much to live for, and the sadness I feel for her having to leave the two main people who really needed her in their lives.

Life is better now, it can be busy but that's ok, and I cannot believe it is nearly the third anniversary of Diana's death. It feels like only yesterday, the memories are as clear as day and will never leave me.

I thank all the people that were involved with us on this extremely difficult journey and being part of our lives, the ones we may never see again will never be forgotten. Rita, Mary, our friends. Jenny and Pat for letting me offload. Amanda, Katherine and the various carers, Jack and his wonderful team, Ellen Diana's counsellor, Sian the speech therapist, Claire, Dr Coles' specialist nurse, the nurses at our medical centre, Mad Hayley, Sue, and Diana's doctor. The solicitor and her secretary, always at the end of the computer to help me, as I bombarded them with emails.

Without all these people life would have been even harder than it was.

James, after applying for many jobs is now working for the same company as his dad, (see not what you know but who you know!!!!) He had an interview, they liked him, and he got the job. Did it help his dad being there? Probably. He did have the first part of the reconstruction and after being very unwell is now recovering from the last part. He has finally got his life back on track. He hopes to one day take that personnel trainer course. He and Louise are still going strong.

John and Chloe had another baby in July 2012, a wonderful little boy they named Robbie after Chloe's deceased dog. All I can say is thank God the dog wasn't called Fido! They have moved to a three bed house and continue to live in organised chaos! I wouldn't have them any other way.

Mark and Kylie have moved to a bigger place and go from strength to strength. Mark made most of the amazing furniture for the house. They are planning their wedding which takes place this August. Olly will no doubt have a brother or sister soon.

Mum is still having regular check-ups, she has been incredible through all this. Her oldest brother sadly died recently, which was very upsetting for her, but she carries on like the trooper she is. God bless her.

Dad has had no ill effects from his aneurysm and rides his bike every day to get his paper and a bit of shopping for Mum. He waits for his next holiday which I'm sure I can arrange again soon!

Adam exercises every day without fail. He has never forgotten that you only have one heart so he is making sure he looks after it! Sadly his mum passed away a few months ago, she will be very much missed. Adam continues to be my rock!

Me: It has taken a long time to write this story, as there were days when I found it too upsetting especially when Diana first passed away, and then of course finding the time to sit here without interruption. I look after Olly every Monday as Kylie has gone back to work and a bit of babysitting here and there for Rianne and Robbie. Having grandchildren has been a blessing and a great distraction. My diet continues!

Liam and Lauren, my little heroes, I hope they are both happier now and settled to their new way of life; they have been a credit to their mother. Lauren has a steady boyfriend and they hope to move in together soon, Liam has had a couple of girlfriends but is yet to find the one; she is out there somewhere! I know they will always miss their mum but hopefully time will heal. As to the future and their father I do not know, that decision will be left to them.

Lauren changes her hairstyles and its colour like a person changes their socks, but it's all part of being a hairdresser.

Liam is still soft, sweet and cuddly and will always need help through his life.

Diana should have been here for all this. God created life, why not let people live it and die old? Life is a lottery, what's round the next corner only God knows (maybe)! They say live each day as your last and how true that is. I feel grateful to be here, whereas I didn't give it a thought before, but Diana's dying so young opened my eyes as to how vulnerable we all are. I am going to enjoy my grandchildren and of course my family as much as I can. I will enjoy every holiday that I take and enjoy every day that I live and be grateful that I am living it. What have I learnt? Patience I think. I didn't have a lot before everything happened. None of my family asked for this so I had to be there to help as best I could.

I wish my family happy and healthy lives. God bless them all.

The End